MW01224689

TANTRIC SEX

"Ever since
that first sexual
experience, even though I
managed to develop what others
might call a healthy sex life, I always
had an underlying sense that there must be
more to sex. What motivated me in my exploration,
and kept me going when I felt discouraged, was that here
and there in my life were scattered moments of love
that were glaringly different from the rest. When
they occurred, time seemed to stop, become
elastic, and the air, the space around
me opened up to reveal a new
dimension of sensual
perception." —D.R.

ESTD 1936   TEL : 23317331
41523058

AMRIT BOOK CO.

Books on India History, Politics, Philosophy, Religion, Yoga,
Ayurveda, Travel, Music, Dance, Astrology, Palmistry,
Children Books, Computer - Management, Hindi Books

21 - N. Conn. Circus Opp. Scindia House, New Delhi-110001.

TANTRIC SEX

A Unique Guide to
Love and Sexual Fulfilment

DIANA RICHARDSON

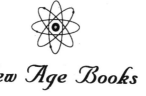

New Age Books

ISBN: 978-81-7822-188-5

Reprint: Delhi, 2007

First Indian Edition: Delhi, 2004

(Originally published in the UK by John Hunt Publishing Ltd.,
46A, West Street, New Alresford, hants SO24 9AU under the title
"The Heart of Tantric Sex")

© 1999 by Diana Richardson

Published by
NEW AGE BOOKS
A-44 Naraina Phase-I
New Delhi-110 028 (INDIA)
Email: nab@vsnl.in
Website: www.newagebooksindia.com

For Sale in Indian Subcontinent Only

Printed in India
at Shri Jainendra Press
A-45 Naraina Phase-I, New Delhi-110 028

CONTENTS

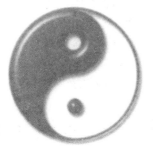

LIST OF FIGURES

INTRODUCTION

THE FIRST TIME I MADE LOVE, I recall being overwhelmed with disappointment, especially since I had waited for love and made it a special occasion. I asked myself, "Is this what all the fuss was about? Surely there must be more to it?"

Ever since that first sexual experience, even though I managed to develop what others might call a healthy sex life, I always had an underlying sense that there must be more to sex—especially since there was such a taboo around it, so many rules and regulations concerning sexual behavior. I always found sex to be enjoyable, but somehow I was never deeply touched. Neither was I as absorbed or as involved as I had imagined I would be.

When I realized that I had made love repeatedly, but still had no real understanding of how sexual energy functioned, I decided to begin a sincere exploration into the mysterious matter of sex. What motivated me in my exploration, and kept me going when I felt discouraged, was that here and there in my life were scattered moments of love that were glaringly different from the rest. When they occurred, time seemed to stop, become elastic, and the air, the space around me opened up to reveal a new dimension of sensual perception. It was as if I was suddenly truly alive and an inner body intelligence took over. I hadn't a clue how and why this happened but it gave me hope that there was something fundamental about sex that I had still to discover.

Today, I know I am not alone. In my extensive work with couples over the years, I have encountered many people facing the same disappointments and asking themselves the same questions. Just like I was, they feel trapped in a cycle which is repeated every time they make love, and rarely involves anything creative or new. Disinterest and boredom eventually creep in. Some will try sexy clothes and videos while many others change partners often to keep sex interesting and exciting. Even so, this seldom satisfies in the long term. While a couple may continue to love each other, the sexual attraction often dies and they stop expressing their love for each other in a physical way. Sooner or later they might even find themselves deciding to separate. And yet for us all the search for this expression of love goes on, generated by a deep longing that seldom goes away.

After researching intensively for many years I discovered that it was the experience of Tantra, that of *relaxing* into the sex energy rather than putting pressure on it, which gave me what I had longed for intuitively throughout my life. It was like finding a series of keys, which opened door upon door. It was a process of uncovering age-old secrets about sexual energy that touched my spirit, bringing me to an unexpected inner peace.

There was a completely new language to learn which slowly became essential to an uplifting experience of sex and love. This language introduced me to a new and different world where the sexual rut disappeared and creativity flourished. I found that many of my ideas about sex were hindering my journey and that to acquire this new language I first had to unlearn the old one. It took me many months to wade through the misunderstandings society had given me, to finally find a relaxed place away from the pressure of orgasm, which I had believed was what sex was all about.

How to keep love fresh and new is the real challenge for lovers today. Indeed, how can we increase this love and make it grow? In its unique and intelligent approach to sex, Tantra offers answers that have the effect of enhancing intimacy and deepening love. Tantra, which removes many tensions from sex by suggesting we relax, surprisingly offers us increased joy and fulfillment. This is what so many of us long for in the deepest parts of ourselves, but we simply don't know how to create it in reality.

I have a friend who was in a dilemma. In love with two women, he was utterly confused, in distress and agony over which one to choose. He went to a therapist, who asked him,

"Who do you enjoy making love with more?"

"Cathy," he said.

"Then go with Cathy," was her advice.

When my friend first told me this story, I was in the doldrums of a long relationship where sex had lost its joy and spark, and I didn't understand his therapist's answer. Now I do. I have learned that whenever sex is fulfilling, the chances of love and a joyful life together are greater. Sexual rapport creates possibilities for intimacy and honesty, and a bonding, loving union. Conversely, where there is dissatisfaction in sex, the seeds of discontent are sown, resentments, frustrations, and fears easily arise, and slowly the love and rapport between partners can break down, ultimately leading to separation.

Our collective lack of knowledge is so acute that it seems like a normal state of affairs for young people to be struggling in ignorance, trying to harness sexual energy, the natural force of life. We pay so dearly for unfortunate sexual experiences or uneducated guesses early on in life, carrying them as swirling, dim, unresolved memories that affect us day by day. Sex, love, and intimacy can become a nightmare ruled by insecurity and lack of trust. Tantra is an ancient art and an antidote, a re-education in sex, and an education that our parents, grandparents, and great-grandparents never had.

Over time, experimenting with Tantra has shown me a new style of lovemaking that has made not only my sex life far more fulfilling, but also my experience of love, and thus life itself has become more significant. Before, I felt I was swimming in shallow waters, unsure of my role in this life, of what to do and how to be. Together with my lover, as we embraced the Tantric teachings, penetrating the deeper waters of sex and the heightened love that arose through it, my life took on a new vision, and I felt as if I was arriving home. Today I can see that the roots of true contentment lie not on the outside of me, but rather *within* me, and sex has become a vehicle for me to contact my core, my inner world, my silent self. It has given me much more depth and substance than my ambitions and achievements ever could.

Tantra reminds us that true relaxation starts with sex. Unfortunately, in our society we have forgotten the art of relaxation in most areas of life. And sex in particular has become a source of anxiety and stress for many of us. We are conditioned with countless fears and tensions around sex, but once we begin to relax *during* the sexual act, we will find that many of our anxieties and unhappinesses naturally subside. If we can relax *into* the sex energy, the inner comfort that it produces will radiate out giving the rest of life that same quality of relaxation and loving ease. In exploring sex we become more intimate with our own body and sexuality and that of our partner, too. With this comes an acceptance of the simple truth, with nothing hidden, that naked is sacred. And out of this arises a confidence based on self-understanding. Through the experience of Tantra, we find that what we have always hoped is true: love and joy can be a tangible reality for each of us, not an impossible dream.

Two primary sources made this dream possible for me. My years of experience and inspiration are based on two audio-tapes entitled "Making Love" produced by Barry Long. In these discourses he offers revolutionary insight into men and women, and a completely different perspective on love and lovemaking. At first, in my ignorance, I was too proud to admit that I did not know, in truth, how to make love. I returned to these teachings some five years later, during which time I felt I had exhausted the routine of sex. But now my attitude had changed. I listened to the tapes in gratitude, knowing there was definitely something I did not yet know about love and sex. The depth and detail of information given by Barry Long changed the course of my life. Through ongoing experimentation within the specific guidelines, I was able to face and challenge my sexual conditioning. This essential groundwork gave me the experience of discovering a new "genital connection." Furthermore, it enabled me to understand and absorb, in a bodily way, the words of my spiritual master, Osho. He includes a vision of spirituality through sex, woven together with interpretations of the ancient Tantric scriptures which were born in India thousands of years ago. These words remain a treasure to humanity today. Both these sources represent Tantric teaching at its highest level.

This book is an attempt to share practical information about sex that created a subtle and significant revolution in my life. It is by no means intended to be a comprehensive presentation of the origins or intricate esoteric aspects of Tantra—it is simply a personal experience. The material appears in three sections: "The Roots" looks at the divine potential of sex and love; "The Love Keys" offers practical body-oriented suggestions; and "The Journey" delves into crucial aspects of sex and sexuality. Sex is a vast subject, and even while attempting to streamline the information, the different themes naturally link and interweave. Reading "The Love Keys" again and again, in conjunction with your own experiences while using them, will bring you deeper insights into sex, support your exploration, and strengthen your perception.

PART
I

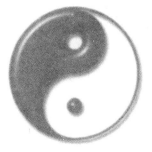

THE
ROOTS

INSPIRATION

T HE MALE BODY AND THE FEMALE BODY ARE SIMILAR, *but still, different in many, many ways. And the difference is always complementary. Whatsoever is positive in the male body will be negative in the female body; and whatsoever is positive in the female body will be negative in the male body. That is why when they meet in deep orgasm, they become one organism. The positive meets the negative, the negative meets the positive, and both become one—one circle of electricity. Hence so much attraction for sex, so much appeal. This appeal is not because man is a sinner or immoral, it is not because the modern world has become too licentious; it is not because of obscene films and literature—it is very deep rooted, very cosmic. The attraction is because both male and female are half circuits, and there is an inherent tendency in existence to transcend whatsoever is incomplete and to become complete. This is one of the ultimate laws—the tendency towards completion. Nature abhors incompleteness, any type of incompleteness. The male is incomplete, the female is incomplete, and they can have only one moment of completion—when their electrical circuits become one, when the two are dissolved. That is why the two most important words in all languages are love and prayer. In love you become one with a single individual; in prayer you become one with the whole cosmos. And love and prayer are similar as far as their inner workings are concerned.*

Osho, Vigyan Bhairav Tantra, Vol. 2, Chapter 27

I

REFRAMING
SEX

EVERYONE IS INTERESTED IN SEX. It is the one
subject that continues to be of undying fascination, if not
obsession, throughout the millennia. You can tell
immediately when sex is the focus of a conversation; heads
move closely together and there is a hushed intensity, a virtual
thickening of the air. But when people are afraid to talk about
sex or ashamed of sex and its "animal" nature, there can be a
palpable feeling of separation, a screen of isolation and tension
surrounding them. The fact remains that whether sex is being
discussed or ignored, repressed or expressed, enjoyed or
endured, it is the single most significant aspect of our lives.

Sex is always in the mind. It forms a central theme in our
thoughts and daydreams. It is part of our chemistry, as each
sentient creature on this planet was created in sex from the
union of male and female cells. Our recognition of this begins
early in childhood when we naturally fondle our genitals with
innocent comforting delight, and our sexuality accompanies us
throughout our lives in various stages of development and
expression. It is the source of a great deal of pain and pleasure,
of comfort and discomfort. It often determines our happiness
and unhappiness, our ecstasies and our agonies.

The simple act of painting our toenails or lips and the

splashing on of perfume or aftershave are steps towards attracting sex. This is highly obvious today when we are constantly saturated with sexual images, words, and films. The media use sex to advertise, to disgrace, to scandalize, and people use it to control, to entice, to abuse and abandon. Our obsession with fashion and appearance has a lot to do with sex. Being seen by someone as attractive gives us vitality and confidence, even if we don't find that person particularly attractive. When desire is shared we see the possibility of love, and this fills us with joy. It is what each of us truly longs for, to love and to be loved. Nothing can take its place. And when we love someone, sex becomes an ongoing means of communication.

Sex can also be the cause of miscommunication, of arguments, violence, confusion, discontent, and restlessness. I've heard it said that men think about sex every three minutes and women think about it every six to seven minutes. Whatever the real statistics, the fact remains that we as human beings are in an ongoing relationship with sex, whether we like it or not.

Sexual energy and the life force

There is simply no way of containing sexual energy; it is the life force itself. Even though in our minds we often try to separate sexual energy and "other" energy, the truth is that it is all one and the same thing. Energy is simply energy with an inherent capacity to move, and it moves, whether the life force expresses itself through sex or survival, in art, athletics, or music. And try as we might, we cannot repress or ignore this energy, we can only learn to channel it in the most intelligent and uplifting ways.

As prevalent as sex is, it is a rare person who has discovered a way to derive full satisfaction or a loving heart from its practice. In inquiring into the phenomenon of orgasm, modern research reveals that an "average" sexually active person experiences orgasmic ecstasy for twenty seconds a week, ninety seconds a month, thus eighteen minutes a year.[1] And this is based on an orgasm lasting ten seconds. Even ten seconds can seem quite an achievement! So in fifty years of sexual activity we have the privilege of experiencing orgasmic ecstasy for about fifteen hours in total. This is astonishing (and distressing) when you consider how many times you make love and how much additional time is spent dreaming about it and agonizing over it!

Obviously, love and sex are not in a satisfactory state for most of us. Sex is not the orgasmic, innocent, spiritual force it is meant to be, transporting us into a world of love and true passion. It does not deeply fulfill us, giving us the strength to face each day with enthusiasm, nor does it have the power to take us beyond the pressures or limitations of our day-to-day life. Sexual problems between men and women are common, such as sexual abuse, frigidity, ambivalence, premature ejaculation, impotence, and sexual disinterest.

Sex and intelligence

In order to reverse this and find the depth of sexual satisfaction we seek, we must begin to bring intelligence into our view of sex. We have to start looking at it within a new framework, to see it from a different perspective. We must look beyond reproduction or immediate physical pleasure and gratification. This new picture will give us fresh insights into sexual energy, how it best responds, and how to utilize sex as an ongoing creation of love between men and women. And the good news is that sex is an extremely healthy and empowering force, which we can enjoy and use to our great benefit.

Sex in its highest form has an element of the divine in it. It brings you to "here," to the divinity of the present moment where you feel gloriously at ease. Everything rests perfectly in place. It is an orgasmic biological ecstasy which arises out of the dynamic interplay of opposite forces, and which is food for the spirit. Sadly, many people of religion hold the opinion that sex is a distraction on the path to God. "Avoid sex at all costs," some of us have been taught, even if you spend your nights dreaming restlessly about it and your days thinking obsessively about it.

This is a great misunderstanding and an aching loss to humanity. If sex is limited to reproduction and instant gratification and its subtle spiritual function is ignored, our life energy is dissipated, disturbing mind, body, and spirit. With Tantra, the cosmic balancing of male and female energies, yin and yang, positive and negative, dynamic and receptive, we can introduce love and spirit in our lives, within and without, and learn to live beyond the limitations of simple biology. We are offered the opportunity to return to our nature as men and women, and to find the spiritual language of love through the physical act of making love. It is a different picture of sex than the one we inherited. Tantra gives us new insights and a completely different vision of sex and its function.

Phases of sexual energy

In human beings, sexual energy is understood to run in a circular path along internal channels through the body, with two distinct phases.

The first phase and initial impetus of sexual energy begins in the brain before circling downward to the genitals *(see* fig. 1). More specifically, the hypothalamic-pituitary region and the pineal gland in the brain secrete hormones that control the endocrine system in the body and these include the sex glands.

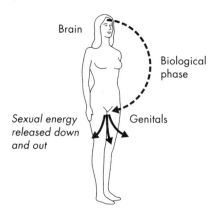

Fig. 1   Biological or reproductive phase of sexual energy

18

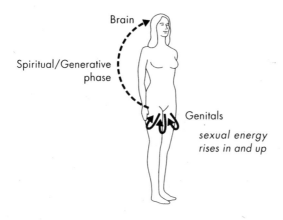

Brain

Spiritual/Generative
phase

Genitals
*sexual energy
rises in and up*

Fig. 2   Spiritual or generative phase of sexual energy

These hormones maintain sexual well-being and promote the eventual readiness for sexual intercourse. This is the first and *descending half* of the circle—from the brain to the genitals. It is known as the biological or reproductive phase of sexual energy. And it is here that we invariably release the sexual energy created in sex, through orgasm or ejaculation.

The secret of Tantra, and its prime interest, is that sexual energy is encouraged to be *retained* in the body. It is not habitually released in orgasm or ejaculation. It remains within the body and is re-circulated, and through this we fulfill our orgasmic potential. In this the second half and *ascending* phase, sexual energy is given the opportunity to circulate back to its source in the brain, so as to revitalize and nourish the "master" glands (pineal and pituitary) in the body. These glands have a profound influence on health. Sexual activity is known to release many hormonal factors that positively affect body and attitude, and since ancient times sex has been associated with longevity and spiritual illumination. When sexual energy can be re-absorbed, recycled, sex becomes a revitalizing, energizing force. This is known as the spiritual or generative phase of sex *(see* fig. 2), and here the genitals are viewed reverently as *generative* organs. Accessing this second phase of our sexual energy by allowing it to turn inward and upward, is the revelation of Tantra. It shows us that sex can be directed to create *more* life, not simply another life.

This spiritual phase of sexual energy arises as men and women learn to relax together during sex. This is contrary to the popular experience of sex as effort, an activity involving tensions and pressures. We believe that the more we *do* in sex, the more will happen and the greater the reward. We hardly think of taking it easy! What we don't realize is that genuine sexual ecstasy goes hand-in-hand with physical relaxation. The more we relax, the more we feel. In fact, ecstasy and tension are diametrically opposed; tension creates heat and restlessness while ecstasy arises from a coolness and an inner peace. Tension narrows and contracts, while relaxation opens and expands. Tension creates a peak, while relaxation creates a valley. Tension forces a release, while relaxation allows absorption.

Relaxation is the whole ambience of Tantra. It means that when we relax down into our sexual energy, instead of building

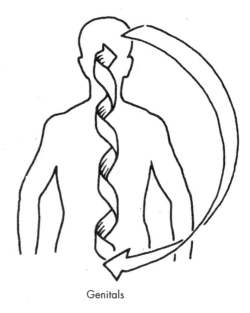

Genitals

Fig. 3　　　Complete sexual energy circle, with redirected sexual energy spiraling through energy centers it up to a peak and then releasing it, the outcome will be more life energy and more love. In re-directing sexual energy through relaxation, we can turn it inward and upward, where it is automatically re-absorbed by the body and re-circulated *(see fig. 3)*. Tantra refers to this step as placing a foot on the first step of the inner ladder of growth. In time, a neglected energy pathway forges its way open in the core of the body, and we experience this from the genitals upward as a streaming electromagnetic current, a glorious golden light phenomenon. When we encourage the spiritual phase of sex instead of obstructing it as we do in our ignorance, lovemaking becomes a sacred experience filled with wonder.

KEY POINTS:

ॐ Sexual energy is the life force itself running through us all.

ॐ By balancing our male and female energies we can enjoy a healthy, empowering sexual relationship.

ॐ We can direct sexual energy in the usual way by orgasm or we can redirect it to give us more energy, more love.

ॐ Sex is transformed creatively into a truly uplifting experience.

Notes

1. The Art of Sexual Ecstasy, Margo Anand, page 347 (quoting from ESO by Alan P Brauer & Donna J. Brauer).
2. Sexual Energy Ecstasy by David & Ellen Ramsdale, pages 118—121.

2

SEXUAL CONDITIONING

IF SEX IS SUCH A NATURAL FORCE intrinsic to all human beings, how did we lose touch with its deeper orgasmic potential? How did we lose the art of generating love? Of staying in love? Why are we so focused on orgasm? The simple answer, sadly, is that as we have become more civilized we have become less conscious. Over thousands of years men and women have fallen dramatically out of balance with each other. We have become progressively time- and goal-oriented, conditions in which true love and uplifting sex deteriorate.

With technological development we have become addicted to time, to achievements, to plans in the future and to reaching our goals, whatever they may be. The more highly developed the country, the more important time becomes, with people living on tight schedules with back-to-back appointments. This creates so much pressure we not only lose our ability to love, we actually become sick. Stress is responsible for an extremely high percentage of illness in the modern world. Relaxation and inner ease have become so unfamiliar to us that when we are not "doing" anything we feel restless and bored. We long for action, excitement, stimulation. It seems that we have reversed the rules of nature. Living with and against the clock seems to give our life meaning while "being" and stillness and quiet arouse our anxiety.

Why are we so goal-oriented in sex?

How often have you said to your lover or yourself, "I want to make love. I just don't have the time." In a sense that is true, because satisfying sex requires time. However, when we do finally make love we are always in a hurry to get to the end part, the orgasm part. When we are striving toward that, we are ahead of ourselves. We are not really "here," we are not even really together. We are almost using each other and our every move or touch is oriented toward our goal. The orgasm has become the only means of fulfillment, and we feel that sex is not really sex unless we "come," unless there is a peak and release of energy. When this is our experience, millions of women are worried, in emotional pain, when the elusive orgasm is not reachable, and most men are deeply concerned because they ejaculate much sooner than they would like—or at least well before they can satisfy their partner. Unless we "come together," we feel that we are missing something, that we have failed or are sexually inadequate.

This urgency for an orgasm operates unconsciously within us, almost like an automatic reflex, seeming to leave us little choice but to head for orgasm, as we usually do. This desire is so strong it seems to be absolutely instinctive, which makes it even harder for us to imagine there might be other ways of making love! And so we repeat ourselves in sex, looking for a certain fulfillment that we never seem to find.

This tendency of goal-orientation, and the resulting haste in sex, has been going on for centuries and together with religious dogma, it has effectively and seriously repressed our sexual energy. We are subject to a host of fears, insecurities, anxieties, tensions, and pressures around orgasm and sex, and our pleasure is kept, through this and unknown to us, within certain definite limits of enjoyment. We have lost knowledge of alternatives in lovemaking, and the expression of our sexual energy has become subject to certain conditions which dictate that we automatically travel along a specific sexual route: we start *this* way and we finish *that* way. It is virtually a routine. And unfortunately these conditions operate without us even knowing they are there, because mother and grandmother and great-grandmother made love in this way and if it was good enough for them, why not me? That is the way I thought until I began exploring love within a different frame.

From doing to being

The eventual outcome is that through forcing the sexual energy toward reaching a specific goal, we have lost the capacity to discover how the genitals themselves "make love"; what they "want to do." We have a fixed idea of what we want in mind. In this way we have unsuspectingly lost our "organic genital intelligence," and today sex is a function of mind instead of true body. This sexual conditioning has led to an extroverted and biological approach to sex. Along with it our sexual energy has become congested and our bodies unduly tense. Our lifetime habit of compressing sexual energy and forcing it intentionally although unconsciously along a fixed, goal-oriented route, has resulted in a chronic twist in sexual energy, with what could be described as an almost "corkscrew" effect. The accumulated physical and emotional tensions of our past experiences sit in the genitals making them tense and much less sensitive than they should be. Sex is now more of a mechanical "doing" and reproductive function and we are without access to the divine "being" aspects of sexual union. We only know how to "do" in love, and not how to "be" in love.

Picture a flower that stays compressed in a bud, restricted, and never given the opportunity to open and blossom. Such is our condition. It is a chronic tension, and the sexual center is turned and twisted in on itself in such a way that the naturally expansive energy is prevented from radiating throughout the body. Sex becomes limited to local genital sensations, we are unable to create higher ecstatic experiences. The inward and upward swing of the sex energy required in Tantra happens as bodies and genitals relax, no longer compelled by orgasm, and that same energy spreads and expands deliciously through the body. Yet very few of us have had this experience because we simply get much too tense as we try to control and force the direction of the sex energy. When the same energy is free to move absolutely of its own accord, sex becomes a glorious mixture of rampant passion and sobering silence.

Personal psychology and programming

The sexual center is the seat of our individual psychologies and personalities. This is where our programming is molded. Our earliest unconscious impressions surrounding sex and life are lodged here, affecting us long before we become sexually active, and on into the rest of our lives. The negative imprints, the centuries of sexual misunderstandings, the phrases, the looks, insinuate themselves into our bodies while we are still young. In this way we inherit our sexual conditioning, which resides in the body in the form of physical tension with a restless, excitable quality. The tension of our collective past adds to the tensions of our personal past, and these can be both conscious and unconscious.

Excitement and sexual tension

As soon as our level of sexual excitement reaches a certain point, the unconscious tension within each of us is triggered to form an urgent physical desire, which sets up a powerful craving for orgasm. With this forceful injection of tension, we swing automatically away from the here and now, working frantically toward an artificial climax created by a focus in the future. In fact we are not truly present in sex because we have gone in pursuit of a specific outcome. In this way sexual energy fails to be an empowering and moving force, but simply a pleasurable build up and corresponding discharge of tension. This sexual tension unfortunately seldom moves through or out of the body completely. Instead, it lives on as frustrated desire, accumulating with time and continually seeking release. It makes our genitals tough and insensitive while it makes us feel emotional, restless, lustful, or angry. When this accumulated tension is triggered, or thrust forward by sexual stimulation, it adds to the already disturbed energy in the sexual center.

Like the foundation of a building, if the base is weak, all the upper structures will lack strength and support from the earth. In the same way, the higher energy centers in the body will also lack vitality, nourishment and integrity. Therefore, when the tensions of achieving orgasm are the underlying theme of lovemaking, an already bottom-weak system will cave in. The pull or corkscrew twist on the fragile sex center will automatically hook and mobilize the entire collective unconscious surrounding sex. When the flood of psychological sicknesses and perversions that have arisen over thousands of years seep through to us today, the innocence and spirituality of the sexual act is lost. This is effectively a psychological sickness, and while it is expressed through the body, it is really a condition of the mind.

Time for relaxation

Tantra directly addresses the mind and the restlessness of the psyche by re-aligning us with our essentially sexual nature. Sex is an aspect of the spirit. Since heart and spirit have little to do with the sexual act today, the recent resurgence of interest in ancient sexual attitudes and practices is a sincere attempt to turn the rising tide of sexual ignorance. By bringing intelligence into sex, by experiencing sexual energy in an innocent, playful, childlike way, absorbed beyond any preoccupation of outcome, we begin to sever our ties with our conditioned personal and collective pasts, and open up to a new world of experience..

To begin, we need to have a flexible attitude toward time because time is what we make of it. If time is money, then time exerts pressure to fit more in and do more things. Where time is cyclic as in nature, there is patience, which removes pressure and replaces it with relaxation. Some plants wait for years for the rains to come so that they can blossom for a few short hours. Have you ever wondered how on earth you would get everything done, then suddenly you are on the plane, up and away, with everything sorted out and slotted into place? If time is what we make it then it must be flexible, where time can even stand still. This happens as we enter the present moment, which is why Tantra asks for an *unhurried* loving approach. When we are not in a hurry, or concerned about time, this makes us aware of the unfolding present moment which is filled with richness. When I lived in India, I observed that time had almost no significance; in fact nobody really cared about it in the slightest. Yesterday, today, tomorrow—it did not make much difference. Interestingly in Hindi, the same word, "kal," is used to describe yesterday and tomorrow! This attitude toward time gave the whole country an extremely relaxing quality, one of being rather than doing. On any given day an overcrowded train can stop, and stand dead still for five hours at the end of a five-hour journey, just twenty minutes from its destination, as mine did without any explanation for the nature or the length of the delay. When this happened to me, the other passengers just sat quietly, there was nothing said or done, and everyone fell into immediate, joyful acceptance. Adults relaxed and chatted, children played and moved about the crowded compartment as if they were at home, spicy snacks appeared and eventually the train started up again. No panic or fuss because no one was determined to reach their destination by any specific time.

After living in India for several years and having returned to Europe, I remember traveling on a German plane from Frankfurt to Berlin. The young businessman next to me kept checking his watch, agitated because the departure was already one minute late! When we took off some fifteen minutes later he was absolutely furious that life's circumstances had interfered with his goal by a few minutes, and he would be late for his all-important meeting. He was restless for the remainder of the journey, unable to experience even a moment of peace and relaxation.

In the Western world, goals, plans and time rule our lives. In fact these days it is almost chic to be busy and often we keep busy to avoid facing the insecurities or anxieties we may feel about love and intimacy. How often have you been too busy for love? And then when you found some time, it was last thing at night, a quick fifteen or twenty minutes before you went to sleep. Or it was a quickie first thing in the morning before work. In this kind of sex, time has entered our lovemaking, and brought with it the pressure that something *has* to happen, and fast! So in our desire to create pleasure quickly, we move immediately toward orgasm because it feels good. In contrast, Tantra tells us that lovemaking needs time, lots and lots of unhurried time. Sexual energy needs hours to relax, blossom and flower, to bring the deepest pleasures of satisfying lovemaking. When we give ourselves this opportunity we find beautifully fresh and unexpected experiences, where the energy itself celebrates differently each time. You cannot possibly get bored. In truth, we ourselves are creating not only the difference, but also the extent to which we are able to relax into the immediacy of the moment.

A healing force

This Tantric dimension opens up naturally and accidentally when lovers are relaxed, open and available to each other, perhaps freshly in love or surrounded by the gorgeous greenery of nature. Many of us have had this magical experience where the moment itself feels like heaven. I remember it happening to me spontaneously in India during an intense monsoon rain, late one night. The thundering and torrential rains created the sensation of being encapsulated within a whirlwind of intensity. I was with my lover of many years in his huge bamboo bed when suddenly time stopped and we moved as one body, passionate and aimless, consciously absorbed in the unfolding present moment. I was golden and floating, ecstatically filled with love for hours, with no idea of how I had gotten there.

Through Tantra I can now access this mysterious present dimension consciously and at will, not merely by accident or chance. Many of our problems, anxieties, and unhappinesses, even illnesses, have their source in sexual issues. When we validate sexuality by incorporating consciousness as nature and God intended, we discover sex to be a healing spiritual force. And surprisingly, the sexual interest does not gradually burn out as is commonly experienced by lovers. In glaring contrast, the attraction *increases*. The sexual experience gets finer and finer as time passes, the genitals learning to respond to each other with a new ecstatic "intelligence."

Tantra, which is everybody's birthright, removes the darkness and brings light to life.

KEY POINTS:

ॐ Tensions of our sexual conditioning block our true orgasmic potential.

ॐ Discover the journey of sex and forget about the end part.

ॐ An unhurried approach creates a quality of timelessness, one of being present.

ॐ Through this the sexual organs re-discover their ecstatic intelligence.

3

POLARITY AND THE POSITIVE POLES OF LOVE

THE GREATEST INSIGHT OF TANTRA, indeed its cornerstone, is that masculine and feminine energies are equal and opposite forces. These attract and complement each other, as do yang and yin, dynamic and receptive, positive and negative (see fig. 4). This signifies that when men and women are joined in sexual union, the bio-energies of the bodies create an ecstatic sexual experience through the interplay of opposite polarities. And this happens without doing anything. In effect, the Tantric journey begins when we contact and re-establish our inherent male and female polarities. This presence of opposing polarities or forces in man and woman is crucial, since it introduces us to a whole new vision of the sex act.

Male and female polarities

Our sexual conditioning has sadly clouded our natural polarity, leaving men and women out of balance with each other. We can imagine the bodies as two magnets, which have the capacity to create an attractive magnetic field in each other's presence. Instead of the poles being shiny and bright in order to respond to each other vibrantly, our poles are smothered in rust, dust

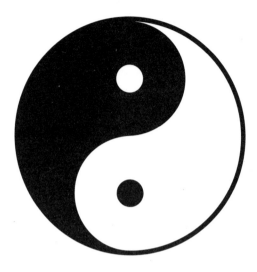

Fig. 4   Yin and Yang symbol of equal and opposite forces

and fuzz, which interferes with the magnetic field and the flow of energy between them. Through our conditioning urging us toward orgasm, it is almost as if we have disturbed the original polarity or charge in our bodies. This cloud of disturbance now veils and obscures the male and female polarities. In other words, the effort and activity that we customarily pour into our lovemaking creates a friction-style heat, almost a screen of "over-charge" that can be likened to static electricity, which disturbs our genitals and makes the sexual energy unable to respond through polarity.

When we make love operating against the inherent polarities of the sex organs, we are unwittingly working against our own ecstatic sexual potential. Through making love *in consciousness*, we are able to purify (decondition) ourselves of this energetic disturbance, and the bodies will gradually and gratefully return to their intrinsic male and female polarities. Men begin to feel their true masculine qualities and women their genuine feminine attributes. We generally are not aware of this falsity or disturbance in our polarities because it has been our sad condition for so long, but what is apparent these days is that women are increasingly tough and manly while a great many men in turn are more macho and aggressive. Both men and women are suffering from the effects of a distressed sexual energy. We were born with this imbalance, and from the first moment we make love, unless we are guided differently, we are reinforcing it.

Re-educating ourselves about sex

There has been so little guidance on sex for centuries. In asking my women clients how much information they were given about menstruation as girls, the answer again and again is none. No information whatsoever. Many were given the appropriate paraphernalia well before the event, and that was it. This is a monthly experience for a woman, inextricably linked to sex and reproduction, yet we receive little or no guidance. As a parent, what do you truthfully know about sex that you could pass on to your son or daughter? Most men and women have received absolutely no information about this core aspect of their lives. I was in the same boat, and once I decided to re-educate myself, it took me quite some time and commitment to regain the sensitivity I had unknowingly lost. I had to learn how to relax and "be here" while making love, rather than be interested in "doing" and going "there" toward orgasm.

The essential step for me was to acknowledge my polarity and fall increasingly into it. I focused on how to become more "negative" and passive, so to speak, more allowing, more receptive, more conscious, and it surprised me to find my man becoming more "positive," more dynamic, more vital, more "here." This was not the same kind of positive I had known formerly, where lovemaking could be described as a pushing hard linear event, creating a peak of energy. It was almost the opposite, like the inverting of a peak, a bottoming out. It was something new and different, deeply touching, circular, ecstatic, unimaginably joyful. Whenever I fell back into my peak and release pattern, I would feel frustrated, irritable, incomplete, and no longer close to my lover.

I slowly learned that this new "style" of lovemaking gave my life meaning, a spiritual quality that I had been searching for in other ways. I felt as if I had arrived at a restful fireside after a long time wandering in the wilderness. I gradually discovered that love was strengthened through an inner focus, rather than an outer focus, and that it depended more on me, and my consciousness, than on him. In this way suddenly everything was back in my own hands, and I began to see that I was entirely responsible for the quality of love in my life. When I made love consciously I noticed that I was much more loving and lovable.

Loving in a magnetic field

Male energy represents positive and female energy the negative, counterparts of a single phenomenon. Each half alone is incomplete; it is only through each other they exist. However, it is important to understand that each polarity, either negative or positive, contains its very own complementary opposite pole (see fig. 4). The man, while essentially positive, also has an inner negative pole (an inner woman), and the woman who is essentially negative, contains a balancing inner positive pole (an inner man).

In this way both are independent of each other, a unit unto themselves, each with an inner positive or negative. This gives each body the potential to create and circulate energy within itself. The male body is carrying the positive pole in the genitals and the negative pole in the chest and heart area. The female, in natural opposition, carries the positive pole in her breasts and heart and the negative pole in her genitals. Between this positive and negative a magnetic field results, and the sexual energy is enabled to stream and spiral upward through the body. This magnetic field between the two opposite poles is called the "rod of magnetism" (*see* fig. 5).

When these two "magnetic rods" are in the presence of each other a powerful magnetic field is created between the bodies. Joined in full-bodied sexual union they are meeting at their opposite poles, an "electrical" circuit is completed. Male energy flows from the penis into the vagina and up toward the

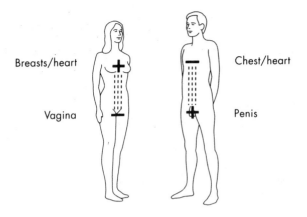

Breasts/heart

Vagina

Chest/heart

Penis

Fig. 5   Male and female bodies showing opposite polarities within
and the rod of magnetism

woman's heart. The female energy responds through the breasts
by penetrating the heart of the man and flowing downward to
his sex center. A complete unit is created and the circulating
bio-energies have the power to generate flickering light. With
this circuit complete the electricity passes back and forth from
man to woman with active and passive phases, man becoming
woman and woman becoming man. It is a divine bio-electricity

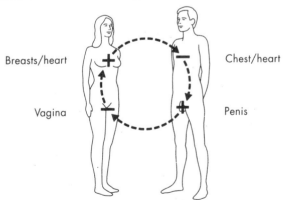

Breasts/heart

Vagina

Chest/heart

Penis

Fig. 6   Circular movement of energy between bodies creates
a "circle of light"

which long preceded the modern invention and Tantra refers to this phenomenon as "the circle of light" *(see* fig. 6). This powerful polarity effect represents the highest potential of man and woman together, as a spiritual force through which it is possible to penetrate the mysteries of life.

This information about polarities must be drawn into our lovemaking in a very practical way. Since body energy flows, not unlike electricity, from positive to negative, it is the *positive* poles of the male and female bodies that need to be awakened to initiate the deeper movement of sexual energy. The importance of this approach is signified by Tantra calling the penis and breasts the "positive poles of love." They are the source of all life, semen from men, milk from women. Treating them as such during foreplay and sex makes all the difference to the quality of sexual energy generated.

Generating sexual energy through polarity

This means in practical terms, that for a woman the breasts are infinitely more important than her vagina. However, our usual approach in lovemaking and foreplay, which consists of touching and stimulation, is to place all the emphasis on both sexual organs. We think about getting these two together as soon as possible, and sex usually proceeds as soon as the man has an erection and well before the woman is sexually awakened. For a man the penis is his positive/dynamic pole and it is ever-ready. However, for a woman, this is her passive/negative/receptive pole, which is not ever-ready. The focus is inadvertently placed on the penis and the vagina, the organs of love, when we should instead be focusing on the positive poles of love. This approach is extremely common, but in terms of female body energy there is a serious misunderstanding, and this ignorance lies at the source of our great dissatisfaction in sex.

Men and women are tremendously frustrated (even enraged) through the inability to generate sexual energy through polarity.

When attention in foreplay is given to a woman's clitoris and genital area it is energetically ineffective even if exciting. She cannot become deeply sexually aflame because her genitals are of secondary importance as far as her inner body polarity is concerned. To invite her bio-energy response, the positive pole, her breasts and nipples must be engaged, and her heart warmed. The love and energy built up here in the positive pole resonates and overflows naturally, showering warmth, receptivity, and willingness into the vagina, thus awakening the passive pole.

The organ of love cannot be ready until the positive pole of love is included in the picture. This true awakening of the vagina introduces what could be described as "electrical potential" between the penis and vagina, when upon penetration (or at any time later) suddenly the male energy floods into the circuit as a thrilling current of life force. It is a completely different experience of sex. When loving emphasis is placed upon her breasts prior to penetration, the readiness for sex is there, both physically and psychologically, and this is very important. The man will immediately sense that the woman is with him, on his side, moving in rhythmic unison. There will be a feeling of oneness with a deep bodily yes from her, and he won't have to fight for his love, or she struggle to give it. It is true sexual union.

Making love in this way, utilizing polarity, begins the process of establishing a powerful energy field between and within two bodies. Bio-electricity flowing within this magnetic field follows a spiral path, and this explains why the movement of the famed serpent power—the kundalini energy, located at the base of the male spine—will be experienced as a forceful unfolding, jerking, rising snake. In complementary style, the root of the female kundalini energy lies not in the spinal base as mistakenly believed, but in the breasts. This is so because energy cannot be raised from a negative center. Once the breasts and heart of a woman are fully resonant, this snake will implode, gracefully unwinding and giving way within. Through the bio-electricities, lovemaking can move to previously unexperienced heights as the energy connects and vibrates deep within the bodies and souls. We are enabled to love passionately as the body electricity takes over, a sense of timelessness pervades, each moment ecstatic and orgasmic, something we may have only dreamed about. Then the delights of lovemaking will grow, since there is no end to polarity, only the possibility of more and more light.

The way to ecstatic sexual union

The art lies in creating and harnessing polarity, and so returning to intrinsic polarities whereby men become more masculine while women become more feminine. Through being able to truly love and satisfy a woman in sex, which represents a man's deepest longing, he begins to feel himself more grounded, mature, responsible, loving, energetic. A genuine male authority and clarity arises. A woman in receiving and returning this love, begins to experience herself as innocent and sweet, the source of love and creation, and a delicate perfumed femininity arises. Falling into balance through this intrinsic polarity creates harmony understanding, respect, and mutual appreciation. Love becomes a living reality. Once we embrace polarity an innate attracting quality develops, an organic magnetic intelligence between the penis and vagina, which strengthens with time. The amazing result is that we require less and less effort to make love; the body does it by itself. Indeed, the less we do and the more we let ourselves be, the greater the experience.

The ancient Tantric symbol, the Shivalingam still found all over India today, depicts the penis or *lingham,* usually surrounded by the vagina, or *yoni.* These are shown in a variety of interesting shapes and forms, but the *yoni* here has far deeper implications than simply representing the negative female pole. It also represents a channel, a highway to the heart through which the man can reach and unite with the female positive, his counterpart. In divine sexual union, the positive male pole penetrates the female negative, reaches upward, ultimately penetrating the heart. When this happens, a kind of golden interlocking effect occurs, the penis encased and absorbed gloriously within the heart. This is pure ecstasy!

KEY POINTS:

ॐ Male and female are attractive forces as are positive and negative.

ॐ This polarity is the source of our sexual ecstasy.

ॐ Each body carries the opposite pole within which forms a "magnetic rod".

ॐ Two bodies in union create a powerful magnetic field and circulate bio-energy.

ॐ To activate the sex energy a woman's breasts must be loved and caressed.

4

AWARENESS OF BODY
AND MIND

THE ART OF TANTRA most simply defined is the union
of sex and meditation. It is simultaneously a physical
and a spiritual happening, where two seemingly
opposite extremes are joined into one. When this happens, a
magical quality arises, and we have the sense of entering a
fourth dimension where the mysteriously engulfing "present
moment" awakens. In this realm everything sparkles and
radiates creating a freshness in the eyes, a song of love in the
heart and a new appreciation of the surroundings, our lover,
and ourselves. We feel highly sensitive and porous because the
essential energy of the Universe, pulsing life itself, is moving
through us.

In conventional sex we do not achieve this sensitivity or
aliveness because we are usually not aware, not conscious of
what is happening. We are simply doing it, often mechanically
or habitually, and hopefully enjoying ourselves, but we are
usually lost in the activity of it. In conscious sex we are
attempting to be aware of what is happening at each moment,
and through this we create the opportunity to have an enriching
experience of love each time. This happens because we
understand the real nature of sexual energy—that awareness
transforms sex into love.

A natural meditation

For this reason Tantra invites us to become aware and conscious of ourselves as we make love. We don't get lost or become mechanical; our attention is inward, we are present to our senses and feelings, we are "here." While making love a natural meditation arises. To most people, meditation implies being alone, sitting upright, still and unmoving, but this is only one form of meditation. The movements in sex need not be chaotic but restful. They can revolve around a core of stillness, as in ballet or tai chi or swimming. Contrary to popular belief, meditation can arise most easily during the sex act because its physically pleasurable intensity helps us, even forces us, into the experience of what is happening as it is happening. This awareness of the unfolding moment creates the experience of "here", one of "being present," from which an inner peace and relaxation arises. This is the sought-after fulfillment of meditation. The mere fact of bringing the consciousness to reside within the body whether we are moving or lying still, creates a silence, depth, and presence. The body can move around and change position as much as it wants, it can even fly, but throughout it all the consciousness remains quiet, still, and serene.

Slowing down and being unhurried during sex to experience the present is the way we can begin to have an experience of consciousness. We must take time to listen and be inwardly attentive to subtleties that rise out of an inner focus or stillness. As a couple continues to make love in this relaxed way, a new level of sensual perception and sensitivity grows with time and familiarity. The experience becomes increasingly pleasurable and ecstatic. In this way sex can become a profound ongoing meditation where communion happens between the bodies and spirits of two people.

When we speak of changing the way we make love, we find that awareness is at the core of it. It is a crucial key to lifting sex to a new height. The first step in awareness is that we must continuously pay attention to our bodies and become aware of precisely what we are doing and feeling as we make love.

Slowly, slowly we become alert to each movement, each gesture, each breath. When we learn to watch everything that is happening inside of our bodies, and *be with it,* the very act of sex becomes our whole focus, or realm of perception. And the very phenomenon of being it and watching it, transforms it.

When we bring awareness into our bodies, we will be surprised to find that it is a world unto itself with many different realities operating simultaneously. The heart is beating, breath is rising and falling, and we can feel certain vibrations, tingling sensations and warmth, even light, through the body. When we become too involved in forms outside of ourselves, their colors or content or character, if our minds are preoccupied with something else or someone else, our

awareness will be diffused and ineffective. Our awareness is also greatly diffused by our interest in orgasm, because in our focus on an event lying ahead, we miss the precious present moment. Even if we are one second ahead of ourselves, we are in fact absent. As we begin to challenge out habit of being absent in sex, we have to begin establishing presence in its place. We have to learn to stay in the here and now in the body, and this requires tremendous awareness.

Focus on the present moment
Sex offers us the opportunity to practice and intensify awareness in order to literally create the present moment. We learn to "be" more in sex, and to "do" less. Out of this the magical Tantric experience emerges. Suddenly when there is no goal, there is an injection of spontaneous and uninhibited life energy. The natural attraction between the penis and vagina is so strong, so full of life, it gives easy access to the present moment.

When we walk, for instance, it is easy to drift off into thought because foot contact with the ground through a shoe is not exactly a heightened feeling (although it can be if you want it to be). Likewise when we cook, the wooden spoon in our hand does not create tremendous delight, no thrill. It is easy for the mind to drift off to other matters. The intensity of sexual union, and its powerfully engaging nature, makes it easier for us to be aware of the elusive present moment, unlike when we are walking or cooking or performing any familiar task. The pleasures of sex with awareness form an experience, the very nature of which can anchor us in the present moment.

Be aware of yourself

To assist us into the present moment, Tantra asks that our attention and awareness be on ourselves. In conventional sex, I have found generally the attention is on the partner first and foremost, as we focus on his or her pleasure. How is he doing? I would ask myself. Does he feel good? Am I doing it right? Is this enough or too much? He was almost more important than me. As I placed my attention on my lover in these and other ways I noticed I did not have a real inner connection to my body, or a sense that I was rooted inward and downward. I was all up and out, and essentially I was making love for somebody else.

Tantra taught me to pull my attention back to myself, to forget about the man and to engage with my own energy first. It taught me to bring the awareness in and downward and back into my body, to feel my belly and my breath, to make love for myself, before I concerned myself with him. This may sound crazy, but it makes all the difference! It creates an ease and relaxation out of which a natural intimacy and attraction arises, and where insecurities dissolve easily. It means that I energize and unite with my own body first, before I join it with another. I bring my body to my lover, inwardly in attunement, alive and joyous, ready to make love. With this attitude of putting yourself into prime focus, rooting and centering yourself inward, so much more can happen in love.

This was initially clarified for me during my practice and teaching of bodywork. Massage is something I have taken great joy in giving throughout most of my life. I decided that I needed to be more qualified, so I learned some new techniques, more advanced and sophisticated, but I found much to my dismay, however, that the spirit and joy of giving disappeared when I focused on a specific outcome. After some time I decided to drop whatever fancy techniques I had learned and returned to the magic of massage in its oily simplicity, cruising down the contours of the body, slipping and sliding along the musculature. I felt the delicious textures, each one an engaging story in itself, while I hunted around for knots and hard sinewy bits. For me, these were always the most "juicy" spots to play with, and I soon forgot to think about *how* I was doing it. Instead I began to put my whole focus on *what* I was touching. How did the body tissues underneath feel? How did the fingertips most enjoy searching? What would feel most delicious if this was me lying here? Where did my hands most want to touch, and how?

I began to forget about the person I was massaging, concentrating only on the movements of my own body, my breathing, my internal relaxation, and the interior of the body beneath my searching hands. I noticed that the more I focused on my body, my hands, the deeper the person seemed to relax, and an almost ringing silence would emanate from the body. They would feel extremely benefited from the massage, deeply rested, at peace and refreshed. They had lost sense of time, an hour of bodiless eternity. The more I focused on myself and the moment, the more the other person was able to relax back into themselves. I remember feeling guilty when I stopped thinking about their physical problems during a session, but whenever I had simply loved touching their bodies, the people always felt better, even enriched. Today I teach my massage students to focus on *themselves* and the innocent joy of touching and giving, to stop worrying about technique and simply to bring love and consciousness into their touch. Technique has value, but the person using the technique is even more valuable.

Relax into your body

In the same way, when we make love we must pull ourselves back into center-stage, focus on and become familiar with the interior of the body, learn to relax all over. When you are relaxed, your partner is more relaxed and vice-versa. The more we relax, the more we become involved in the present moment, and from here the sexual experience can emerge spontaneously. The intensity of turning the awareness inward onto the delicacy of the genitals during sexual union encourages consciousness to awaken in the body. The body then becomes a temple and sex a god-given meditation.

Our new approach is essentially a shift from mind to body, so I suggest couples forget about each other, their personalities or problems, and focus on their inner world. When I was retraining myself this approach worked well for me, allowing my mind to slip into the background, and the body was an anchor that created my inner reality. Because senses and sensuality are greatly enhanced through awareness, and because love is made in the physical body, we must learn to expand our sensory awareness, its feelings and perceptions. What is happening in our very own bodies? And where? Remember it is a matter of pulling your attention from the periphery to the core, from the outside focus of the mind to an inside focus of the body. What am I feeling and where am I feeling it? How does it actually feel? Exactly where do I feel the awakening of life in my body? Where is the light in here? I often suggest to couples at the beginning of a workshop to look around inside their bodies "for a place that feels like home, a root."

When you find such space, be with it and rest. Give it some light or color; vizualize making it bigger. Get a sense of it as a location in the body where you can root yourself and find some peace. It may be the belly, the heart, genitals, lower back, anywhere, but not the head! Wherever it is, hold it in your awareness, and grow into the feeling of it. Remember, you can *return home any time* you find you have suddenly walked out of the front door, and you will find this happens often! We have to continually step back to our inside space, leaving the outside space outside. It is as if we literally have to step inside our bodies, create the inside space and keep expanding it. The outside space is usually much bigger in people than the inside space, so we have to "force" the boundaries of the inside space open, to expand.

At the outset of lovemaking, when each person gives the time and attention to his or her own body *first*, by expanding their inside space, it is as if the air between the bodies that normally separates them actually comes alive, like a magnetic field. You become aware of the life in your own body which radiates outward to communicate with the body and presence of your lover right through the space between you.

The perception or inner awareness of the body is a far more delicate phenomenon than the thinking process. When our attention is caught up with thought, it is difficult to reach down into the vastness of the body to experience what is specifically happening there. It is difficult to "be" in the body. One contributing factor is that at the outset of making love, we are much too fast in bringing our bodies into physical contact. We compress what could otherwise be a prolonged and wonderful exchange into a few seconds flat, trying to create something enjoyable for the other. This has the effect of pulling each person out of awareness, off center, and away from home. Rather than feeling ourselves by dropping inward and absorbing the other, being sweet and simple, we put more effort into doing something to them, a rub, a touch, a caress. We have become human "doings" and forgotten how to be human beings.

Let your body be your guide
To experiment with this slow approach, try this exercise:

EXERCISE

Before you make love, lie in bed on your sides and face each other, your bodies slightly apart and without any physical contact. Pull your focus away from your partner into your own body. Close your eyes for a few moments and feel yourself withdrawing your awareness from the outer to the inner. You can imagine you are sliding down your own spine vertebra by vertebra, into the back, down into the pelvis, and so connecting with the energy in the base of your body and legs. Hold yourself in there for a while, and give yourself time. This brings vitality to your own body before you bring your bodies together. After several minutes, open your eyes and look at each other. As this happens you keep your awareness in your own body. Breathe. Relax your jaw. After a few minutes, slowly, slowly inch forward toward your lover keeping your focus inside. Move into an embrace, the slower the better, starting with a meeting of the fingertips, and let it be more of a "happening" than a "doing." Be acutely aware of each body part, the skin, the warmth, as it meets and wraps itself around the other. If you wait long enough just "being," you will find the bodies are eventually pulled or sucked together, attracted like magnets. Remove any intention, and be with the experience of moving closer to the one you love. When we move into love with this slow sensitivity, awareness of ourselves and of our partner is greatly expanded. The body energies too respond vibrantly to this languid lazy approach.

You can also try this when you are greeting each other after a separation. Before you hug, stop, stand still and take several seconds to draw your awareness inward, ground yourself in your body, your legs and feet. Then step forward as slowly as possible and move into a gradual hug with your lover. Stay relaxed, drop your shoulders, don't make any undue physical effort, breathe. With awareness stay in the body, let the *bodies* do the greeting, and allow it to be a melting together.

Pulling the awareness inward in this way, instead of projecting it out, creates a more sensitive environment within the body. You become aware of places that you didn't know had feeling or sensitivity, because your attention was placed elsewhere. And while making love our attention is frequently preoccupied by thoughts of orgasm. When you can be present in your body, you begin to experience your dimensionality, an exquisite interior between your front and back that explodes into sensitivity like an inner display of fireworks.

Switch off your mind

We are diverting the focus from our periphery to our core, from an outward expression to an inward impression, and thereby enhancing sensitivity in the body. Tantra returns us from sexuality to sex. Today we experience our sexuality rather than the true force of sex, because the mind has become an integral part of the sex act. To return to the innocent and natural state of sex we have to start by switching off or disassociating from the thinking part within.

Perhaps the biggest distraction in sex today is the incredible ability of the mind to fantasize. Indeed, sexual fantasy has become the driving force of many people's sex lives. Often in lovemaking we get involved in sexual fantasy, not conscious of what is happening in the present. Our attention is not on this partner here and now, but on creating an imagined one or an imaginary situation. Thus we are not really experiencing the truth of the body. Instead the mind is using fantasy to drive or motivate the body. Sexual fantasy can be habitual, as if we are repeating the same program again and again.

Almost every one of us I am sure has used a sexual image, either real or imagined, to help us get excited and maintain an interest in the sex act. Mostly we use sexual fantasy to urge us toward orgasm because the imagination helps us to reach the peak. It works incredibly well! The mind must be proclaimed as a powerful tool to produce such effective, even immediate results. But sexual fantasy is, nonetheless, a great diversion as it pulls us away from reality and the person we are making love with right now.

Tantra, in its wisdom, embraces this imaginative power of the mind. It encourages it to be re-directed into the body. The imagination can be harnessed to actually stimulate valuable movements of energy within the body instead. And this happens because sooner or later the energy will follow the imagination. We have all tried it, and we know it works. Imagination can thus be used as a positive tool in sex rather than a distraction. For example, if we begin to imagine light and circles of energy within the body, or energetic connections between the positive and negative poles (inside and outside yourself), or energy streaming from a man into a woman, or a woman absorbing this golden light, or energy radiating from the heart and breasts or leaping from the penis, sooner or later we will begin to have the feeling of this actually happening. The energy can be imagined as a streaming golden flow or even a jumping, leaping of light, even lightning. Men may find this works easier for them.

A return to innocence

It might be indistinct at first, but your awareness will help to fan it, and this makes energy grow and expand. Some people "feel energy" more easily than others do. If it is not easy for you, please use your imagination; it is a tremendous support to the body. Where you do have the sensation of energy moving within, the imagination can help to intensify the experience. In these ways the mind is used to pave the pathways for the inner energy circuits, which become more and more dynamic as time passes.

In the transition of sexuality to sex, the returning of sex to the innocence of the body, we must remind ourselves that the first step is to be aware of the inner music of the body, and the second step is to be aware of the thoughts. Even if we are not using fantasy in the sex act, we are often thinking all kinds of thoughts, and these thoughts are potentially destructive. When we become aware of our thoughts, estimated at about 50,000 per day, it is a surprise to find out what else is going on inside of us. In my early sexual life, when the kind of lovemaking I had been longing for was actually happening, I noticed with horror that I would find myself drifting off and thinking about something else. I was astounded that it could be something as banal as where to go for dinner! I found it difficult to be utterly involved in sex. Since then I have discovered that sexual energy is so subtle and sensitive, even one sudden and simple thought is enough to disturb its natural magnetic flow.

A gradual process

When we are bringing awareness to our thought process, it is not as if we must stop thinking. We can't! We do think and that is the problem! There is nothing we can do directly about thinking, however, we can approach it indirectly. The significant thing is to notice that you are thinking, caught up in a stream of thoughts, and in that very noticing you are thrown back into the present, you sever the thread to the thoughts. By simply acknowledging that you were thinking, you disassociate or "cur with the mind." This is enough, and you return to the present. Do not begin an inner dialogue giving yourself a hard time because you were absent and not present, simply and quickly slip back into the present. Stay immersed in the present, in the physicality and sensuality of consciousness in the body, until you find yourself caught up in thinking again! Notice, and slip back into your body immediately.

It is a process, and the miracle of the phenomenon of awareness is that you need not do anything except to become aware. The simple act of watching your thoughts, becoming aware of the physical patterns associated with them, will bring about a change. The mind becomes more relaxed, content and attuned to the body as if a bridge is created.

As couples embark on the Tantric journey, it is important to bear in mind that it is a gradual process. It is a shift in consciousness, neither a sudden change nor a technique. You can't do it, you have to *be* it. It is an ongoing refining process of creating stillness, which requires time. It is helpful if you do not seek big changes or immediate results. It does not happen like that every time. Real change is made up of numerous, sometimes invisible, small changes which take root in the body. Notice the smaller, less obvious things that happen to you, what

51

you feel, where you feel it, and the joy of it. This consciousness brought to the body and the sexual act begins to transform it, becoming a fountainhead of love, enriching to body, mind, and spirit.

KEY POINTS:

୧୬ Awareness of mind and body transforms the sexual experience into love.

୧୬ Shift the awareness from outside to inside.

୧୬ This focus creates a "root" within the body.

୧୬ Challenge thinking by consciously experiencing bodily sensations.

୧୬ Use power of imagination to amplify and expand energy movement.

5

PENETRATING
INNOCENCE:
THE LOVE KEYS

IN CONVENTIONAL SEX, we can liken our bodies to an open blossom with petals extending outward, reaching out into the world. The energy is primarily projected away from the center, we are each focused on the other.

Learning to live through the body

In Tantra the blossom is consciously inverted, the petals are pulled back toward the center and inverted toward the core as if returning to a bud again. The energy is primarily projected toward our own center. The Love Keys knock us back inside to be focused on ourselves, our inside space, which we consciously have to create and expand. The Love Keys help to draw our attention in from the periphery to the core enabling us to focus the awareness within the body. By rooting the consciousness in the body, and using the body as a constant reference point, we are able to stay increasingly in the present moment. Indeed the body is the only thing that exists in the present moment, and learning to live through the body increases our chances of overall happiness. We forsake the entangled, tortured, drifting mind in favor of the simple god-given pleasure of the flesh.

Polarity, the underlying theme of Tantra whereby the genitals generate an energy of their own, begins to emerge of its own accord as we make love consciously, particularly if we make love consciously *consistently*. With the information about polarity, and the importance of engaging the positive poles (which can be called the background Love Key), the Love Keys will make the body a vehicle, an anchor and a bridge to keep us rooted in the sexual present. The Love Keys will guide us to various parts of the body which open up doorways to being "here and now" in the present moment.

These Love Keys assisted me thousands of times and as I dropped into them, layer by layer, I was slowly able to center my awareness in my own body and thereby regain trust in myself. As a result of bringing consciousness into the act, old sexual wounds moved out of the body, repressed energy was freed up, and I was enabled to shift to a higher frequency. When I first introduced the Love Keys to my experimental group of Westerners while living in India, I was stunned at the dramatically fast response. Love was in the air sparkling in the eyes of both the men and the women! What had taken me years to unravel and rearrange in myself was happening in a handful of days. It was a miracle.

This was reassuring for me because it confirmed that our bodies respond instinctively in similar ways. In working with couples since then, I have established that they can be in their teens or in their sixties, together for one night or thirty-two years, the response is the same. Love flourishes with consciousness. But it must be stressed that establishing "the present" through the Love Keys, and *in the body,* is an ongoing process. It never really ends. Although there can be an immediate sense of an enchanting quality at first, and a more relaxed approach to sex, it takes time for the sexual present to be rooted firmly in the body. You can't expect to be operating one way for several decades, focused on fantasy or the sexual reward of orgasm, and then suddenly move into a whole new way of being.

Moving away from old patterns

As a couple it is very important to realize that changing our lovemaking is an art, it's a journey and not an instant affair. It is made up of small steps, which can sometimes be huge in effect. But the more we experiment with the Love Keys, the more we can practice moving away from our ingrained patterns into the experience of what is happening now. It is a practice of returning to the body again and again. Sometimes we manage and sometimes we don't. Sometimes we will get caught up in the desire for orgasm, and (please) go for it and thoroughly enjoy it. And at the same time be aware that this is what is happening, we are choosing it. This is a great step in itself. It brings awareness to the process we are involved in, and with practice, when we are able to remain present in the body during lovemaking, no longer motivated to do, but happy to be, the body regains its inherent sensitivity and consciousness.

The Love Keys will strengthen your rapport with your lover and a new intimacy will grow. It will be like developing a new language, a solid foundation for love. The awareness encouraged by the Love Keys will allow you to relax and have more time to focus on what is happening inside your body, and particularly between the penis and vagina. As the sensitivity of the genitals increases, and polarity gradually becomes established, the positive and negative poles begin responding to each other, vibrating gloriously. Sex returns itself to the body, and ceases to have anything to do with the mind.

Take the time to create stillness

But this is not immediate. When you approach a new way of sensing the genitals, it may be difficult to feel anything at all at first. It might even be an effort to try and feel. Until this point we have always depended upon a lot of friction for our sexual experience, but now we are searching for a sensitivity that lies beneath this superficial sensation. You are getting in touch with a finer layer, vibrant and glowing, more satisfying. And although you never lose your capacity to become excited, you are moving beyond the initial intensity and overwhelming nature of this excitement. It is almost like stepping underneath it. You must slow down in both body and mind, creating enough stillness to feel something so subtle it has previously been barely discernible. Developing this degree of sensitivity takes time and commitment, but it is so well worth it.

When you begin using the Love Keys, you will feel exposed, vulnerable, a little bit shaky perhaps. This is natural because you are *penetrating your own innocence*. It is as if returning to that childlike wide-eyed innocent state, present and playful, now starting to make love for the first time. It is fresh landscape with different colors. If you feel uncomfortable, embarrassed or a little bit silly, it is fine to laugh. Many times I have burst into fits of wild, uncontrollable laughter, and I always felt so much better, more alive and relaxed afterwards. If you feel sad, allow the tears to flow, be grateful for them, don't hold them back. Laughter and tears are a release of withheld inner tensions, and allowing them expression enables you to relax into a deeper, more authentic layer of yourself, a prerequisite for intimacy and satisfying lovemaking.

Let this be a form of play where we are sincere and not serious. And there is a world between these two. Sincerity arises from the heart, while seriousness arises from the mind. Sincerity likes to experiment and learn, while seriousness likes a foolproof recipe. Playing around with the Love Keys is a bit like peeling an onion. There is always another layer to penetrate, another step inward to the glory of relaxation in the body. When you and your lover are able to be easy and experiment with each other, playfully and willingly with commitment, love is able to penetrate you deeply. You will eventually find that you can create love through your consciousness, that love is in your very own hands, and is not some wild wind blowing through and over you beyond your conscious control.

Explore and experiment

We need a fresh attitude and a loving approach in order to experiment with sex. As a couple we must be curious enough to challenge our usual tendencies in lovemaking, which means we will probably have to give up things that up to now we may have enjoyed tremendously. Since for most of us sex has become a relatively mechanical orgasm-hunting experience—and people will often admit that the excitement of it is not unlike an addiction—we will need to support each other in breaking or releasing the mechanical or doing aspects of sex. But if we remain focused on the usual goodies in sex, and what we are giving up, it will be difficult to see what we are gaining. Often there is a gap between the letting go and the gaining, so we need the patience and willingness to abandon the old ways, and a playful, honest approach to prepare for the new. With this commitment to exploration and the unexpected, it is most helpful when both partners embrace similar attitudes, making ultimate cooperation and discovery possible.

For instance, in the throes of sexual heat and excitement it may be a challenge to stay open to experimentation. You might suddenly experience the overwhelming urge to go for orgasm. And in these moments, nothing seems more important! However, if your partner can help you in bringing yourself back to "now", suddenly the possibility for you to relax arises and in taking the enormous step of dropping beneath this compulsive urge, the mystery of sex will begin to unfold before you. In this way the support and awareness of your partner is essential in order to grow in love, to bring clarity to the sexual experience. When couples make love in the spirit of cooperation, they are helping each other, teaching and learning from each other, and through each other. Together they uncover the path of relaxation in sex. It is not possible alone. When one partner again and again undermines the efforts of the other, stepping away from our unconscious sexual aspects becomes a near impossibility. Without mutual willingness it will be very difficult to explore new terrain.

Right from the start there must be an attitude of vulnerability, the humble acknowledgment that neither of you really knows much about making love even though you have probably done it thousands of times. A woman I worked with introduced herself by saying she had made love at least three and a half thousand times in the same way, and she was here to see what else was possible! If either partner is unwilling to explore new territory, by challenging old patterns in sex, this can lead to a lack of vulnerability. If you think that you *know* what it takes to make love and how this mysterious energy works, there will be no space for different, possibly more refined and sustaining experiences. Instead, you must be willing to acknowledge all of your feelings and to expose your insecurities and fears about sex. If you are too set in your ways of thinking, the higher orgasmic potential of sex cannot be realized.

Banish rules from the bedroom

We must remember that there are absolutely no rules about how to make love. Using the Love Keys is more a question of awareness. Through awareness we are able to discover and learn, we teach ourselves, but rules are imposed on us and sooner or later imply rebellion. It is the undermining tendency of the mind to make ideas fixed and rigid, especially when we feel insecure about not knowing what may happen next. If you have to do something it is not the same as discovering its value through experimentation. "That really works for me," is different from "I must." It is very easy for a woman to become rule-oriented because she is usually the less demonstrative partner physically, so less doing is easier initially. I have seen all too often a woman imposing rules and literally pointing an angry accusing finger at her lover, rather than exposing her own vulnerability in the situation. The man, feeling chastised and with his ego threatened, will react by rebelling or withdrawing his cooperation.

When insecurities appear in a fresh new sexual way, Tantra offers suggestions rather than rules. Try this, we can say to ourselves, and when we do, we gain concrete experience and so we are able to create new guidelines and orientations. We are two people working together in a unit, like scientists with insatiable curiosity slicing through the misunderstandings of centuries. Patience, love, respect, and understanding are the ways of Tantra.

Choosing which Love Keys to try

In Part 2, the Love Keys are assembled under nine general headings: Eyes, Breath, Communication, Genital Consciousness, Touch, Relaxation, Soft Penetration, Deep Penetration, and Rotating Positions. Each of the Love Keys assists us in accessing the present moment through the body. As you read the individual Love Keys you will find there are keys within keys. Each Love Key gives a range of practical suggestions that can immediately be incorporated into lovemaking. There is a lot to absorb so do not think you have to use all the Love Keys all the time and get overwhelmed. Instead, see which keys you respond to as you read, which feel right, which arouse your curiosity. And then start with these. As you begin to feel grounded in each of these, you can begin to incorporate new ones. Also, after a time of experimenting, it will probably make more sense, you will understand more, or find interest in things that did not previously attract you in the slightest.

It is a unique dance, a journey, an adventure. As you experiment your experience will deepen, and with it your perception. Even if you embrace any two Love Keys to start with, for instance, maintaining eye contact and breathing deep and slow, you are most likely to experience a qualitative change in your lovemaking. So you do not have to embrace everything all at once, it is up to you to choose. Besides, it is a process that takes time, remembering that a shift in consciousness, and not a sudden change, is afoot.

I remember a couple telling me, a year after their first workshop, that they had experimented a great deal with the Love Keys but still they enjoyed having the orgasms. The Love Keys enabled them to be more present and loving, and extend the time of lovemaking, which was wonderful, and then just to finish it off they would have an orgasm like a little whipped cream, so to speak. They continued their exploration, attending another workshop during this time. Then two and half years from our initial meeting, the woman suddenly said to me on the telephone, "Do you know, *neither* of us is interested in orgasm any more! It's unbelievable, because it used to be *so* important. But now we have slowly discovered how to be here, it is so much nicer, more relaxing, why bother with orgasms! And we are so happy, so in love."

The beauty is that once consciousness is brought into the sexual act, a process is set in motion and the old habits or patterns slowly work themselves out of the system. New experiences happen and consciousness takes root. So while you are making love, do not be afraid of trying out some of the Love Keys. Just try one or two and see what happens. If you are in a couple and you decide to experiment, you can discuss which to try at first. Often when both partners are using the same Love Keys, say combining positive poles and breathing, the effect on the sexual energy can be strengthened, but this is not essential.

Even if you don't decide beforehand, or you do not have a fixed sexual partner with whom to experiment, you may suddenly feel inclined or inspired to try something out. It can surprise you. A friend of mine in a workshop, upon hearing that the Love Key relaxation also included relaxation of the vaginal muscles, did not quite believe it. She said nothing at the time, but later while experimenting with her lover, she remembered this suggestion, and saying to herself "okay, let it go!" she consciously released her vagina. As it widened and opened the penis instantaneously dived into the depths of the vagina, pushing and probing upward, almost grateful with delight.

As you choose a particular Love Key to play with, keep spreading the awareness through the *whole* body. For example, if you choose to focus on your positive pole, don't become over-focused on the area. Don't let it obscure everything else so that it becomes a concentration or a fixation and thus a tension, instead of a melting relaxation into your body. If you find yourself thinking about it too much then relax the brain, imagine it fanning open and spreading wide. Sweep the body with your awareness, from head to toe and back again, connecting the parts with the whole. This spreads and expands the sexual energy, bringing the body into one organic unity.

How the Love Keys will help you change your relationship for the better

To help us shed the tough layer of our insensitive uneducated past, Tantra suggests three ways that we can explore our sexuality to effectively cleanse or de-condition ourselves of unconscious sexual patterns which affect the quality of love in our lives. The Love Keys will assist you in this. The first is to challenge the habit of going for orgasms. Also notice that we are basically absent and ahead, and therefore relatively unconscious, when we do go for it. The second is to make a shift from doing to being in sex. Notice too that even if we are not interested in orgasm per se, we feel nonetheless driven to do something in order to have a sexual experience. The third is to restore our original genital sensitivity (magnetic intelligence) through relaxation and consciousness of the present moment.

This is an interdependent process. The more you challenge your patterns, the more easily the genital sensitivity is re-established. The more awareness you place on your intrinsic genital intelligence, the easier it is to change your patterns. Some days you might focus on one aspect, some days on another, and some days focus on all at once. It is a complete re-education in sex that happens through making love and not simply by mental understanding. With the practice of relaxing into the sexual energy, and learning to "be," many old emotional patterns, habits, reactions, and problems cease to be motivated. The thrust toward unconsciousness and the energy it consumes is gradually retraced into the silver thread of consciousness weaving in the body.

KEY POINTS:

ॐ The Love Keys strengthen rapport with your lover.

ॐ Curiosity and the spirit of cooperation are vital keys to exploration.

ॐ Expand your "inside space" through immediate bodily sensitivity.

ॐ Let your experience teach and guide you.

ॐ A shift in consciousness is a gradual process of unveiling sexual ecstasy.

PART
2

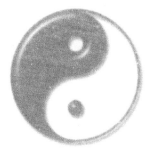

THE
LOVE
KEYS

6

THE EYES

THE EYES ARE ENORMOUSLY SEXY. Often when they meet another's eyes, you will find the surge of sex within you. If you have ever had the opportunity to lie beside your lover simply meeting each other through the eyes, it can be an enormous turn-on and an important part of foreplay. This is because the eyes are powerful channels for sexual energy. They reveal our nakedness and our innocence and expose us to the reality of the present moment. This helps us to be authentic. With eyes open we know where we are and who we are with.

When this channel through the eyes is opened, sexual exchange with your partner becomes more dynamic and vital. It is understood that 80 percent of our energy is projected out of the eyes in normal vision, thrown out and released in looking out through them. This tension is easy to see in people as a lack of structural alignment, where the head and ears lie unnaturally well forward of the shoulders. The eyes, however, are designed to receive an image and we can see without making any effort to see. It happens anyway. The eye absorbs the picture. This implies that we lose, or leak, a great deal of energy out of the eyes in looking. It happens in our daily lives, as we continually search around the environment, keeping an eye on what is happening, interesting distractions, some novelty somewhere, one step ahead of ourselves. Our eyes are more related to the mind and its restlessness, while there is no relationship whatsoever between our vision and the inner dimensions of the body.

Making and keeping eye contact

So, too, in lovemaking. At first when I started to keep my eyes open, meeting the eyes of my lover, I felt awkward and shy, so exposed that I recall laughing in my nervousness and embarrassment. I felt so completely artificial. I could as easily have cried, with the painful revelation that I had never truly been "here" before, been genuine before. I had been accustomed to making love either with my eyes closed or in the dark, and not really available to my lover here and now. But after a short while of experimenting I got used to it, and open eyes soon became an essential energetic connection to myself and my lover. Without it, I felt curiously absent.

In our society we are often reluctant to look someone straight in the eye. We speak to each other while we look around and away, at the mouth, at their shoes, their hair, the baby. Seldom do we hold each other's eyes for a few seconds or longer. We sometimes even interpret eye contact as an intrusion, an invasion of our privacy, or a challenge and exertion of power or authority.

Even if maintaining eye contact while making love feels uncomfortable at first, I encourage you to stay with it because there is so much to be gained. It is the most wonderful sharing of energy and you will often feel an immediate sexual response within you. Eye contact has also helped me to create presence in my lovemaking by recognizing the masks of my personality. After I had laughed and wept my way through them, I felt a freshness and it seemed there was less haze covering the picture around me. A natural intimacy arose, a feeling of closeness, and the sense of isolation dissolved. Then I began to try and receive my partner through my eyes, taking him within my body as I deepened my relaxation. Whenever I reached a point where I felt that open eyes were hindering the consciousness in my vagina, I closed them in order to look deep down into·by body with my inner eye.

Seeing and being seen

Making eye contact is an art in itself. I found it useful to begin by allowing my eyes to have what can be called "soft vision." This means that I allowed everything in through my eyes, a receptive quality. In normal vision we are looking from in to out, but you can consciously switch this phenomenon and try looking from out to in as though the world is looking at you through your own eyes. Like windows, they are simply here and open, receiving. The rays of sunlight shine through the window and into the room. The world penetrates you through your eyes and into your body. You allow everything in your vision to come into you through your eyes, and they become receptive, soft and inviting. When your eyes meet those of your lover, when you look at each other softly and lovingly, you are allowing yourself to be seen. This contact, the awareness of the immediate, brings you quickly into the present moment, and you are here, making love with your partner, rooted in the experience.

There is a simple way to practice this on your own. Go to a park and look at a tree. Don't just glance at it, really look. Appreciate the leaves, the green, the aliveness. Now close your eyes and relax for a while. When you open them again, imagine that you are no longer looking at the tree but the tree *is looking at you,* and invite it into you, through your eyes. See how deeply you can allow the green livingness to enter you. Absorb it into the cells of your body. Then try it with the open blue sky, a puffy cloud, a glorious sunset. Allow yourself to be seen and penetrated by nature. Notice how this practice intensifies your awareness, dissolves your boundaries, increases your sense of connectedness to the rest of the world.

Now, with enough light in the room to see, look at your lover's eyes softly. Choose the eye with which you feel the most natural and at ease. Allow yourself to "be" and be seen. Receive the energy through your eyes, taking it into your body. Invite your lover into yourself, through the eyes. In fact you are receiving the backflow of your own energy, and when this energy is inverted it falls back on the heart, filling and expanding it. It also resonates in the third eye. Now spend time with the other eye. Notice the different qualities in the right and left eyes, the varying colors and configurations. Which eye challenges you more? Which one is softer? Which one awakens the sexual response in you? Stay with each eye for a while and learn to feel comfortable with both of them. Don't flicker back and forth rapidly from one eye to the other. This can be disconcerting for your lover. It can happen if either of you is nervous, so help each other to relax, perhaps by stroking or caressing. To be unsure at this stage is very natural. Do what you can to release any feelings of pressure. Give each other a chance to close your eyes peacefully, and just breathe deeply for a while.

It is important not to stare at the other, since this creates a sense of strangeness, of separation, not one of closeness or contact. The idea is not to scrutinize someone, but rather to allow the other in, and let yourself to be seen. When you stare, you have no presence behind your eyes; you are merely using your will. Blink, be natural, be personal. Don't work too hard thinking you have to keep your eyes open at all times. You may even find it impractical to keep your eyes open when the body positions are such that your eyes are not in easy range of those of your lover.

Close your eyes if you need to

As a general guideline, *make eye contact when you can and when you can't, don't.* Sometimes it is necessary to realign with yourself, with your center, by closing your eyes and feeling exactly what is happening inside the body. The point is not about keeping the eyes open; it is about using the eyes as a way of being here, more available and present. Feel free to close them at any time when you feel discomforted or sleepy, or when you need to be with yourself for a few minutes. When you do choose to close your eyes in this way, it is important to communicate this to your partner, so he or she is not left in confusion, wondering where you have gone.

Remember that using the eyes is only a key to support you,

not to undermine you. If opening your eyes makes you feel so awkward that your body seems miles away, it's better to close them and feel comfortable with yourself. When you feel rooted in your body again, then try opening your eyes again and see how it feels. If you find your eyes burning or weeping, this indicates a great deal of tension held in the eyes. Don't worry; it will pass as your eyes begin to relax with the sensation of being exposed. Always experiment and find the way that works best for you. Hold your faces apart at a distance that feels comfortable to both of you. Some people have difficulties with focus at close range. Expressing honestly what feels right and what doesn't can help you to relax, create the present and become aware of what is happening now.

Holding the space between you

I found that if I faced my partner, made love face to face, it helped me enormously to be present. This sounds obvious because with eye contact we *are* facing each other, but it is more subtle than this. By "facing" I mean allow your faces to be in ongoing proximity, inches apart, with an awareness of the closeness of your partner's face to your face. Use this when eye contact is not possible and also generally when you need a rest from direct eye contact. The eyes can hold the space between the faces, absorbing the skin, the chin, the cheeks, brows, forehead, profile. This brings incredible sensuality into love. I noticed in contrast, that when I nuzzled my face into the neck, shoulder, or chest of my partner I was dramatically less present. It felt familiar and comforting, but it was not a challenge, so easy for me to drift away. The instant I drew back into physical alignment, bringing my head and spine into one line, my face in close range of my lover's face, the effect of regaining consciousness was wonderful as presence entered the air. I found that when I crossed the mid-line of his body, leaned forward beyond his ear, moving my face away from his, or turning my face to the side, I lost contact to this moment. Because of the familiarity and associations of a certain way of embracing it is possible to lose presence, simply because we are accustomed to the embrace. Use the eyes to bridge the gap between you, bringing heightened sensuality as consciousness filters through the body.

Give yourself plenty of time and space to experiment with the eyes rather than make rules, and to receive the sincerity and openness of your lover. See how soft you can become and how deeply you can take him in through your eyes. Look right back into yourself and see how far you can go. One day a moment will arise when a doorway opens and the sex center and eyes unite. It's breathtaking!

KEY POINTS:

ह≃ Eyes are windows of the soul, a powerful channel for sex energy.

ह≃ Eye contact intensifies awareness of the present moment.

ह≃ "Soft vision" makes you receptive, open, brings intimacy.

ह≃ Close the eyes at times too; keep looking inward and downward.

7

THE BREATH

REMEMBER TO BREATHE! Breathe deeply and slowly. When you really get the knack of enjoying breathing, it becomes absolutely divine. It brings sensuality and sensitivity to the body and propels us into the experience of the present moment. Thus breath can be used consciously as a tremendous contribution to lovemaking and foreplay. There are many therapies and approaches to breath that suggest specific and special breath techniques, systems to follow, energy centers on which to focus, where to breathe in and out, but I found it best to just keep it simple, to remember to breathe. When I tried to focus on a specific breathing pattern, I noticed I was focused on the in and out of it all. My attention was riveted on the mastering of a breath technique while my body sensations, the experience of receiving and absorbing the breath, faded into the background. Instead of trying to control your breathing, it is far better as a starting point to simply be aware of the breath in the way that it moves naturally in and out of you.

The breath can be described as a bridge between mind and body, and paying attention to its rhythm becomes a significant anchor to the present. It helps to make a shift from thinking to feeling. If you have ever been fortunate enough to immerse yourself in your breathing you will have noticed that you were detached from your mind. You might even say that you lost your mind, you lost all reason, you were consumed by vital energy and joy of life. This is because breathing unhooks us from our thought processes or the mental element of sex, and connects us with our essential life energy. We begin to feel more sensitive, sensual, and tactile as we make love. Connecting with the breath and consciously absorbing it enables us to reach in between and around our cells, to bring a sense of delicate porousness into the body.

Breathing and sexual vitality

As children, the action of our natural breathing massages the sex center. The easy flowing breath of a baby creates a wave that passes through to the lower stomach and pelvic area. It pulsates through the elastic diaphragm that separates the chest and abdomen, pushes downward on the organs and so pulses into the floor of the pelvis. Here an intricate web of muscles form the genitals, and this acts like a diaphragm which expands out with each breath, continually massaging the sexual center. As we get older our tensions, repressions, guilt, and embarrassments associated with sex, genitals, or masturbation disturb our childlike breath. Gradually, the boundary of the breath moves higher and higher until the breath ceases to reach through the diaphragm to the genitals, or even to the belly. Most adults are breathing into only the top part of their lungs, thus limiting the full benefits of breath. This physical tension takes us away from our deeper breathing to a superficial breathing pattern, holding the fear of vulnerability and receptivity as a barrier. The genitals then lack the vitality and nourishment of the downward inward-flowing breath which pulses continuously into them.

Hence the significance of reconnecting the breath, belly, and genitals during lovemaking. Relaxation of the entire front and mid-line of the body from the throat, heart, solar plexus down to the low belly and genitals, creates receptivity and vulnerability. You are in immediate contact with the environment, noticing the elusive pungent fragrances of the night, the unexpected joyful bird calls and the welcoming damp cool of an early morning breeze.

It is surprising how out of touch with the breath most people

72

are. We breathe without any awareness of the breathing process itself even though our very life is dependent on it. In my first massage session, my therapist kept reminding me to breathe. It was so infuriating. When I couldn't stand it a moment longer, I shouted out in anger how much I hated to breathe. So when I began exploring Tantra, I was not a breath enthusiast. But as I began to change the way I made love and bring awareness to my breathing, I began to breathe slowly and deeply. I noticed after a few months that the restriction was softening, the breath was pushing downward closer to my belly and pelvis. It seemed to be creating its own channel toward the genitals. The more awareness I brought to my breath the more I enjoyed the act of breathing. And the more I recognized breathing as an internal life-enhancing massage, the more I wanted to breathe!

Any awareness you bring to your breathing before making love will make an enormous difference. It may be as simple as being aware of your breath boundary in the shower as you prepare yourself for lovemaking. I noticed that when I was expecting my lover I ran around until the last second, making myself and my home more outwardly inviting. When I began to take five or ten minutes before he arrived to lie down and breathe consciously, I was far more able to welcome him into a pool of tranquillity. Breathing had created receptivity in my body, a femininity that produced a remarkable attractiveness between us.

Breathing into love

Before making love, it is beneficial if you sit quietly for a while, as in meditation where the awareness is turned inward. Even ten or fifteen minutes is enough. These moments of stillness will give you an opportunity to attune to your body and enter into the present moment. As you sit, either alone or with your lover, close your eyes and pull your attention inward and downward. Feel your breathing, and breathe into the diaphragm. You can also imagine the breath following a circular route in the body starting from the genitals up the spine, over the head and down the front to the genitals. When you focus on your breath, you are energizing and sensitizing your inner environment, which will activate your sex energy as you move into lovemaking.

The wondrous life-affirming phenomenon of the breath during sex increases presence, ecstasy, and pleasure dramatically. Breathe in such a way that you can hear your own breathing flowing in and out. This helps you focus on your breath more easily, and your partner is able to hear it too. In this way breath can also become a way of speaking, of communing with each other. It sometimes happens that your partner and you spontaneously fall into a harmonious breathing rhythm together, in at the same time, out at the same time. This will feel superb, breathing the glorious present moment.

It is possible to make a conscious effort to breathe in this way together, which we can call "simultaneous breathing." Listen to your lover's breath and start to tune into his or her breathing rhythm, and begin breathing out and in together. Be relaxed so as to create rapport, not tension, and this will awaken the sex energy. Whatever you try with breathing, it is always important to not make it an *effort*. If you worry about whether you should be having an in or an out breath, or whether you are in harmony or not, you will revert to your mind and miss the experience of your *own* breath. Remember, your consciousness of the breath itself and not the act of doing it will make the difference.

Forming one breathing body

Another way of breathing which we can call "synchronous breathing" may arise during lovemaking too, where one partner breathes in while the other breathes out. The breath moves in a kind of circle and it has a profound influence on the sex energy. This breathing happens very naturally when two people are deeply merged in sexual union. It penetrates your core as two form one breathing body in profound empathy. To breathe intentionally in this way, however, takes some mental effort, and can take you away from the immediacy of the moment. But try it for fun anyway, and see what happens. Keep the breathing deep and slow. If you like, once you have the rhythm of this synchronous breathing established, you can then enhance it by imagining a circular route for the energies. The man breathes in through his heart and out of his penis. The woman breathes in through her vagina and out through her heart. Imagine the breath to be golden light as it moves around in a circle. This can be particularly beautiful when the lovers are sitting up together, the woman's legs embracing the pelvis of her man. This intimate exchange where the chest and breasts meet enhances the experience of polarity within the bodies.

Although breathing through the nose is more refined as it affects the meditative and subtle body centers, mouth breathing may help you to be more fully aware in the body. Breathing through the mouth affects the lower body centers and the emotions, so feel free to use whichever style of breath works for you in the moment. If you are having trouble "being here," distracted or upset about something else perhaps, I would recommend breathing through the mouth, since it can be useful to clear the emotions, which otherwise limit sensitivity and presence. If you or your partner are swallowing a lot, it usually indicates that an emotion of some kind is on the rise, and the swallowing is an unconscious attempt at repressing it. If you feel the urge to swallow, try to relax into *not* swallowing, allowing the repressed energy to move up and out. It takes quite some effort to resist the reflex to swallow, but it is well worth it. You may find that some laughter or tears, or even strong coughing lies beneath the reflex action, and allowing this expression brings you into contact with your sexual energy at a deeper level.

Playing with your breathing

As you begin to bring your breath into focus, it is easiest to start with an out-breath first. Expel all the air from the chest, really force it out. Hold your lungs empty for a few seconds, then relax, and the breath will arrive forcefully to expand your chest in a wonderful in-breath. This brings instant consciousness to breath. The physical inrush of it gives an immediate experience of the vitality of the breath, and helps to connect with the flow inward and outward. Do this a few times if you like, and breathe deeply and slowly in a nice steady rhythm. Usually, as we get excited in sex and move toward orgasm and ejaculation, the breath will become shorter and faster, so breathing in the opposite way, deeply and slowly, will create a relaxed environment for the sexual energy. Tantra says that when lovers remain in rhythmic breathing in unison, there will be no ejaculation. If the breath is in rhythm, the body absorbs the energy; it never throws it out.

You can also breathe in with a sniff, sniff, sniff from time to time. The entire in-breath can be made up of many short sniffs until the breath is complete. Wait a moment and feel the life-giving force of the retained breath. Then exhale. A series of short sniffing breaths helps intensify the feeling of the breath entering the body, and also focuses the awareness in the third eye. Have some fun and experiment. Imagine the breath penetrating your body, wrapping around each cell. Intensify the experience by looking into each other's eyes while you breathe. However you decide to play with the breath, make it creative and interesting for yourself. But always remember to feel the breath and keep breathing into the boundary of it. Breathing into the lungs, between the cells, imagine the blood absorbing the oxygen and bringing more life.

When you make love in the deepest relaxation, consciousness merged with breath, the breath gets lighter, delicate and quiet, and may actually stop momentarily. You breathe and the breath does not turn again. If this occurs, there is nothing wrong; it is a wondrous and silent moment. No outward flow of energy is happening, so the breath is not needed. Remain suspended, embraced by the arms of no-time, and just be in this paradise. The breathing will start up again of its own accord and the sexual energy will receive an unexpected kick, surging upward and coursing ecstatically through the inner bodily channels. You and your lover will be merged with the force of life itself.

KEY POINTS:

ॐ Breath has a profound influence on sexual energy.

ॐ Breathe slowly and deeply while making love.

ॐ Breathe downward through the diaphragm toward the genitals.

ॐ Awareness of the breath creates the experience of the present moment.

8

COMMUNICATION

L OVERS OFTEN COME TO SEE ME in distress, not necessarily because the sex is difficult, but because communication is a disaster. They are suffering from so many misunderstandings and arguments. Events from the past, old arguments and issues, continually disturb the precious present moment. They tell me that they haven't made love for days or weeks because they have been busy blaming each other, trying to determine who is right and who is wrong, who is controlling whom, and they have ended up in an exhausted delirium. Ultimately they fall asleep in each other's arms, grateful for a respite before they wake up and begin again.

How to express your feelings

The truth is that some people are naturally good at saying what they feel when they feel it. Others are not even sure what they feel, let alone when they are feeling it, and they can't seem to share their most obscure inner feelings. When emotions are high, words may seem inadequate if they form at all. Whether or not a person is skilled at communicating, most people agree that sharing and being straightforward is a delicate matter. It may involve saying something that seems against the person you love, that a certain caress did not feel good, or wasn't the right thing at that particular moment. The question is, how do we communicate this information without hurting our lover's feelings, without appearing to criticize or to control? This can easily happen because we are all basically insecure in sex. The defenses of the ego can quickly come between you, creating separation and arguments rather than love.

It is essential to be honest and truthful. You will find the truth has a liberating effect on your own energy, and you become flooded with vitality. Be aware to select your words carefully so as to communicate with rather than offend your partner. A good way to start is by saying the words: "I feel..." and keep talking about yourself. Avoid talking about them and what they did. If the result of your lover's touch is a withdrawal in your body, it is often your cumulative past painful experiences related to sex to which you are reacting, and it has not *only* to do with your present partner. Well, in a small way perhaps, but often the overload from the past is causing the reaction. It is probably not the first time it has happened. So you have to be acutely conscious of this as you speak, making sure you are not getting revenge for all the people who ever handled you badly *(see* chapters 22 and 23). For instance, many times I tried to please a man by engaging in a particular foreplay technique which I knew closed down my sexual energy rather than expanding it, but it never paid off. Whenever I tried to work against the truth of my body, I ended up feeling undernourished or loveless. Or I made love with less consciousness than I desired, producing the same undernourished result. It would be easy to blame my lover for not satisfying me, not doing the right thing, while the root cause was my lack of honesty and integrity, my fear of communicating the truth about what I really liked. He was not to blame for my unhappiness—I was!

Communication is a powerful key while making love. Through speaking about what is happening to you *as you make love* you begin to root yourself firmly in your body and this sexual experience, by bringing inner body sensations into the foreground. We are contacting reality through the body, and thereby creating the present moment. Communication supports a shift from mind to body, from thinking to feeling, from doing to being. Through the focus on reality within the body, its differing feelings and sensations, we are able to shift away from the restless mind, its thoughts and emotions. Many of us are so caught up in thinking that we have very little awareness of or within the body, so communication is essential. Share with your partner what you feel *in your body,* where your feel it, and when you feel it. If you do so, you will find yourself becoming miraculously alive, sensitive, and present.

Sharing your present moment

Unfortunately, people rarely speak to each other sincerely about their present moment, especially when making love. It would solve many problems if we did. Indeed some couples come to realize that they never talk like this with each other in daily life, let alone in love. They begin to notice they are always drifting between planning, some distant memory, vague future wishes. When I started to communicate about the present while making love I found it difficult to *speak out loud,* and was extremely resistant at first, but I soon discovered that the resistance was my fear of looking inside myself. I was afraid of being vulnerable, of his judgments of me. I was also afraid to express my joy, afraid of saying how thrilled I was by this privilege, our delicious body smells, the beauty glistening in his eyes, the supple smooth silky skin, the love I could feel emanating from his penis. The more I practiced, as with most things, the easier it became. It was a relief to speak freely. As I shared my truth with my lover a great deal of energy was freed up and my body became more vital. I gained information about our genitals, our bodies, our sensitivities and pleasures, pains, and insecurities. Sharing what is happening *as* it happens creates intimacy and unquestioning openness, which helps you to remain rooted in the body, aware and present together, where love thrives.

I would suggest that you tell your lover what you feel in your body, or heart, and be specific whenever you can. Don't hide anything. Continue a slow dialogue as you are making love, telling each other what is going on inside you, with relaxed pauses in between. The general idea is that in keeping track of *now* and *now* and *now* we create tremendous awareness of what is happening. And this changes the whole quality of the experience. It brings life and consciousness to it. Avoid prolonged or awkward silences to stop yourself drifting away. Use words to bring yourself and each other into the present. I call this "sharing your now". This establishes an honest basis between you, and gives a new-found freedom. It is not a confession, but simple words to articulate truthfully different feelings within your own body. This increases your awareness, intensifies sensitivity and the body energy will expand accordingly.

Feelings in your body

One of the hardest things for me to admit was that when I stopped being so physically active in lovemaking, I could feel very little in my vagina. I was so used to feeling the pleasures of friction that the finer, more delicate ecstatic function or sensitivity was not yet available to me. I felt that I was dead inside, and it was a ghastly moment when I had to confess to my lover that I could not feel myself, let alone him! With this admission I experienced a tremendous sadness and pain overwhelm me, tears emerged with a great deal of sobbing, and with this release of withheld energy, I suddenly and unexpectedly felt more alive in my vagina. A layer of fear and tension that I had not realized was there had actually lifted off my vaginal tissue. I was alive after all and I burst out laughing! Never feel too ashamed to admit what is happening to you. In fact, if there is some shame lurking around, let it be a hint to you that it is a matter for sharing.

In communicating and "sharing your now" as you make love, two significant things happen. First, you are creating the present through the body, a new basis for the sexual experience, and getting to know the genitals (and each other) afresh. And second, and significantly, you are setting up a channel of communication between your brain and your genitals. Through speaking out loud, "what is," it is brought into consciousness, and it is as if that part of the brain controlling the consciousness can literally "hear" your words. By reinforcing the truth and acknowledging reality, the genitals will respond *instantly* with thrilling sensitivity, more consciousness. In this way you are creating the roots of a new sexual intelligence.

Talk about all of it

As you practice, you will find a way to communicate so that your lover is given positive information about how your body responds and opens up. We are all similar, but also individual. There may be things that you like after you are already warmed up, but often too much stimulus initially can lead to a style of lovemaking that is hot and orgasm-oriented. Or the stimulation reduces your sensitivity. Slow down as you approach one another. Take time to sense your own body, and that of your lover too. Ask them what they like, and how they like it. Share too, simply and sweetly, the how and where of touching you. Take their hand in your hand, show them what works best for you. Talk about all of it. And definitely talk to each other about your lovemaking experiences while you are not making love, because this is a tremendous support to the consciousness, and besides, it's the most juicy subject.

EXERCISE

To practice this type of communication for intensifying body awareness and the present moment, here is a simple exercise you can do together:

Lie down comfortably and several inches apart, face each other and make eye contact. Tune into your own body for some moments and be aware of the proximity of your partner's body at the same time. After a few minutes begin to speak, and as much as possible remain with sensations *in the body*. Identify different sensations or bodily perceptions and then speak about them. First let the woman say what she is feeling in her body. It might be a pounding heart, a vibration in the belly, or perhaps a repeating thought or fear. Then the man can say what is happening to him, his body, his penis, his breathing. Only talk about what is happening *now* in heart or body. Don't start a conversation and don't ask many questions. Pay attention to the body and seek your present moment there, then describe it to your partner. Alternate speaking in this way for some time, sharing the now of your body. Keep it simple and direct, without long pauses or silences. Body sensations keep changing, so be aware of them. Don't try to understand or analyze with the mind. For instance, if your partner says they feel some fear, don't get into a discussion about the whys and wherefores. Through this you step away from the intensity of the moment, the reality. Just keep sharing with your partner what you are feeling, and where. Be specific and be sincere and don't try to pretend something is happening if it isn't. Don't talk about something already gone, or something that happened last time. Stay with now. After some time you may notice your body energy becoming more dynamic and a feeling of physical attraction arises. If you continue this kind of relaxed verbal rapport, lovemaking will be a spontaneous outcome.

Releasing fear and tension

When you can do it, it is best to share your emotions and feelings at the moment they are actually happening. If you delay, the energetic intensity and its hidden potential is lost. When you talk about it later it will be like giving someone a news report of what happened, simply another story without the vigor of life behind it. For example, if you are feeling insecure and are able to say to your lover, "I am afraid to relax, I am terrified that nothing will happen," you will discover that the very admission to the fear of nothing happening in sex will have a profound effect on you. You may start breathing fast, tears welling up in your eyes, feel panicky or in pain as you have the overwhelming realization that you have always been afraid. It has always been there unconsciously, a tremendous tension in you. But you did not realize before because you were ahead of yourself, less "here." Now with consciousness or presence introduced into the sexual act through communication and other ways, the restrictive fear is released from the energy system in a cellular way, and eliminated as a toxin that is often reflected in the pungent body odor emitted during such occasions. The intensity of such an experience of the truth changes reality, it is ultimately relaxing. Fears gradually diminish and love grows in its place. If however, you spoke about your fear later, it would fail to have any transforming effects on you. I have missed many an opportunity to reveal myself to the one I loved, choosing to stay in the fear of showing my deepest feelings. But I soon found that I was denying myself more life and joy, and my fear of exposure was an illusion. Speaking up and taking risks brought me only closer to myself and to my lover.

When I am innocent and able to share what I am truly feeling, my entire body and breath come alive. My body responds to my courage and the truth, it vibrates, it pulsates, it trembles. This makes me experience my aliveness, and realize that I am not really being vulnerable to another but rather to myself. Each time I have had the guts to expose my obscure hidden feelings, I was the one that flowered and sparkled afterward, not my lover. He was certainly touched, and it helped him to be more vulnerable too, but I was the one who benefited. Each exposure was like removing a layer revealing myself to me. I finally came to understand that my lover is not responsible for my expansion, my inner growth, my love. Rather, I am responsible for myself, and it is all dependent on me. My own vulnerability and attitude gives me life and sensitivity; it is not the work of my lover that does it. I learned that in order to get closer to my lover I had to get closer to myself first. In this way we can see how much love we are willing to allow into our lives. The more the mask of the personality is challenged and dissolved, the deeper the experience of Tantric union.

The sounds and silence of your body

There may be moments when you are so immersed in the silence and brilliance of the present moment, the intensity of sensitivity within, that it seems virtually impossible to pull yourself up and out from these blissful depths to speak. If this happens to you there is no need to force yourself to find words. Keep relaxing into the serenity and stillness. However, words are not the only way we can use our voices. Sounds in sex are great, and you can use them too, to convey your pleasure. Be alert to avoid sounds that come from the mind and not from the body. This easily happens in sex when we make sounds to please the other, sounds to make it seem like we're having a good time. These are not true sexual sounds. A deeply sexual sound will have a ringing authenticity to it that engages you, and a mind sound is more likely to have a tinny, superficial hollowness. Allow sounds to emerge from your body to express your inner bodily feelings, the ecstasy and joy. Make an attempt to link the sound with the actual feeling inside of you, get the sound to vibrate from within it. It is as if the feeling itself is emitting the sound vibrating and amplifying through you, so deep is your throat in your body. Sound and sex are one.

KEY POINTS:

꿍 Communication is crucial; be conscious of what you say, and how you say it.

꿍 Share what you feel in body and heart as you experience it.

꿍 Words bring immediate consciousness to bodies in the present.

꿍 This gives new information about each other, body responses, a fresh foundation for love.

꿍 To take a step closer to the other, you have to take a step closer to yourself first.

9

GENITAL CONSCIOUSNESS

HAVING CONSCIOUSNESS IN THE GENITALS
means to enter the living part of yourself from within.
In normal sex, we focus our attention outward on the
genitals while we make love, holding it there with intensity in
order to experience sexual pleasure. But in truth we tend to be
unaware of what is really happening to us, usually caught up in
an idea of what we think we want, and using the penis and
vagina to get it.

In Tantra, we don't exactly concentrate on the genitals, we
relax into them. Remember, it is an easy approach and not a
forced or tense one. Instead we bring our awareness *into* them,
and begin to get an inner sense and impression of them. This
internal focus brings awareness into the sexual act and
gradually builds consciousness into the penis or vagina.
Imagining a fire or liquid warmth that fills the pelvic area,
melting and softening the genitals, can be a helpful image. Our
orientation is inward, and by holding the genitals in awareness,
almost listening to them as we make love, we start to see and
experience them, not ourselves, as the makers of love.

Slowing it all down nicely
Slowing down all the movements during sex will naturally bring

genital consciousness as it enables you to feel the genital interaction. At first, this may seem contradictory as you wonder how your penis or vagina can perceive anything without the friction to which we are so accustomed. To slow down or stop moving may seem a bit daunting, or confusing. But as you slow down, you will soon find more genital consciousness and a tremendously deep level of pleasure as the sensitivity is increased. With a great deal of movement there is too much happening to feel the finer genital function.

The first penetration creates the world in which you will make love together, so penetrate as slowly as you can, taking several long moments to feel the yielding softness, the opening and the giving way of the vagina. Feel the whole glorious phenomenon, penetration and being penetrated. There is nothing like it! And then gradually dive into the welcoming depths. This could take several minutes. Once you get to the end, be still and wait. After a while you may want to move out slowly and come in again slowly, or simply remain for a while without moving. Immerse yourself in the sensation of being embraced by the vagina. Visualize your penis as a generator of love energy and channel this into your partner. From this type of relaxed, slow, conscious initial greeting by the genitals, fluidity and sensitivity grows and the sexual act has an effortless quality. With no goals each sexual moment becomes a world of love unto itself.

The more a woman moves her pelvis back and forth, the less sensitive the vagina, and the greater the defense that is automatically set up within the vaginal walls. As a woman approaches orgasm, particularly clitoral orgasm, she will usually begin to move more rapidly, increasing the friction, and it is here that she begins to separate her consciousness from her vagina. If she is observant she can notice that the entire musculature of the vagina is contracted and tense as she thrusts and moves her pelvis to create pleasure. Stated simply, the more contracted the environment, the less sensitive and receptive the vagina. At this moment, when the sensitivity of the vagina should be at its utmost, the complementary female genitals are unable to truly absorb energy from the penis.

Staying sensitive

When women stop the pelvic motion, we can sink inward and retrain the muscles and membranes of the vagina, and thereby the penis, to become more soft and sensitive. Through this we are able to establish genital consciousness. When first experimenting with this, my lover and I would ask ourselves, "How slow is slow?" With me relaxing and he moving one millimeter at a time, I was re-orienting my vagina to feel the event of penetration, the opening, the surrender, the receptivity. It was glorious! He was learning to feel the penetration, the divine warm welcoming sensation. For the man, it can be a bit of a Catch-22 at first. Moving is a hard-earned habit, one that he has always considered responsible for sexual satisfaction, his partner's and his own. For some men this is an easy habit to change while for others, it isn't. It takes practice. But when a man can slow down for a while, if he can simply be in the vagina and relax into the gap of no-feeling, it will be well worth it. Lost sensitivity will be slowly and surely regained. As he switches his focus to other perceptions besides that of friction, he will eventually feel like he is entering an electrical socket, or a highly magnetized environment. It is riveting!

Make love for yourself

The essential step in rooting your consciousness in the genitals is to invert your focus. Place your attention on yourself first and foremost. This means that instead of projecting outward, making love for your lover, you pull in, making love for yourself. As we im-press the energy rather than ex-pressing it, it slides down and back into the base of the body. It is useful to imagine your energy falling back, tracking down vertebra by vertebra into the pelvis. Suddenly we can see and feel the spine as a highway that connects with the genitals, flowing upward.

When we bring consciousness to the vagina, most women will find they unconsciously hold their vaginas tightened and flexed while making love. Many women also consciously squeeze and tighten the vagina believing this will create more pleasure for the man. Today there are even exercises for the vagina which women practice to increase agility and strength of the musculature. This comes from a common fear that the vagina may be too loose, even big, perhaps having been stretched in childbirth, and therefore less interesting. Both the fear and the belief are misconceptions that have arisen out of the use of friction to create sexual pleasure.

If, however, couples choose to experiment with Tantra, perceptive and conscious genitals are essential. It will take some time to regain the sensitivity of the vagina and penis at this deeper level, but if the woman constantly keeps her awareness in the vagina, and remains relaxed, receptivity is increased and a greater energy exchange occurs. The sense of welcoming that is imparted to the vagina through consciousness increases trust and creates the basis for true ecstasy in sex. A serene and conscious vaginal environment also naturally prolongs the sex act. In the same way for the man, it is important that he brings awareness to the buttocks and relaxes his anus, noticing perhaps his tendency to squeeze it tightly.

Tension in the anus is associated with insecurity, and men's fear of not getting or maintaining an erection. Tightening the anus will not allay the fear. It will distort a man's energy as he pushes his genitals and pelvic structure forward, so compressing his sexual experience by confining his genital consciousness. By relaxing the anus the whole floor of the pelvis will soften, the sexual energy can fall down and backward into the body so to speak, and he will feel more rooted in the base of the penis. I have heard this feeling described by men as making love from "behind" the penis, and many have found this to be a most significant Love Key, as it helped to increase sensitivity in the penis and prolong intercourse.

Be aware of your pelvic floor

Most people are completely unaware of the pelvic floor, where it is and what it does. One man in my couples workshop commented that until three days earlier, he didn't even know he had a pelvic floor. Now, he couldn't stop feeling how tense it was. The truth is that we rarely feel all the way down into the tissue of our genitals, not really. Only when we are actually engaged in sex or masturbation do we allow ourselves to feel "down there," and even then only a little. Unknown to us, we are in the chronic habit of holding ourselves *away* from the genitals. We are always unconsciously holding our sex centers very tight. We are tightening the musculature of the pelvic floor, thereby holding the genitals in ongoing corkscrew tension as described in chapter 2 on Sexual Conditioning. This tension also inhibits the pulsing effect of the breath into the pelvic floor.

This web of muscle spreads across the base of the pelvis, attaches to the sitz (buttock) bones, pubic bone, and coccyx and forms the delightful base of the torso. It is these interlacing muscles into which the genitals are enmeshed and out of which they are created. There are muscles that can be used to consciously squeeze the anus tight, and another group of muscles that can interrupt the flow of urine and contract the vagina or make flicking movements of the penis. The pelvic floor also has a central point called the perineum, lying in front of the anus, behind the vagina or root of the penis. The musculature pulls up parachute-like, into a central knotty tendon, which you can feel with your hand when you tighten up. A lump will become palpable under your touch. It is here in particular that our tensions accumulate, spreading down and affecting the energy and structure of the legs and feet. We are continually pulling the floor of the abdomen up. Any time you put your awareness in your pelvic floor you will discover you can relax it and in releasing it, the musculature may drop down two to three centimeters!

The prime characteristic of the pelvic floor is that we are always holding it tight, pulled up and contracted. And we are absolutely unconscious of this central tension. Since I discovered my pelvic floor at least fifteen years ago, it has been a constant reference point. I started taking my awareness to my pelvic floor and *every* time I would find I was holding it tense. I would consciously release it, my body would take a huge sigh of relief, and I would feel more at ease, with my legs and feet having more contact to the earth. Moments or minutes later I would travel there again to find that it was tight! Regardless of how many times I consciously let go, the second my awareness was absent, my unconsciousness, my fear and tension around sex would pull upward to create a tightening. I remember it exasperating me particularly at one time, so I asked a close friend of mine if she felt any tension in her pelvic floor "No," she said "Never!" This was a shock for me! Was I really so tense? More than most? It was some years later we met again, and almost the first thing she said was: "I haven't stopped feeling my pelvic floor since I last saw you! I did not realize that I had never been conscious of it."

Expand the muscles of your pelvic floor

While you are making love, simply relax your pelvic floor to help your genital consciousness. First of all identify it while standing. Pull up all the muscles around your genitals and anus, imagining you are stopping the flow of urine. It's easy. Squeeze a little tighter, exaggerate the tightness. Contract the musculature . . . and then let it go, relax. Imagine that you are bottoming out, emptying out through the vagina or penis and anus. Let the energy flow down the legs. Feel the new inner sensations that come with this. Try this out and then do it as often as possible. Do it anywhere, waiting in a line, while chatting at a cocktail party, it's okay—nobody can see you, and it feels great! Suddenly you will find yourself more at ease, more confident with a sense of belonging. Make this an awareness exercise that you do again and again because it brings vitality to the pelvic area. But do not do it mechanically or unconsciously, otherwise it makes the vagina tougher. Feel instead that you are keeping it in tone, balance the pulling up with the releasing down, do it slowly millimeter by millimeter and see how the consciousness grows. The beauty of awareness is that it knows no bounds. Women can always find another layer of perception in the vagina by forcing the consciousness into the vagina and asking themselves, "Can I be more open?" Miraculously the musculature will widen a few millimeters, and as the very cells are penetrated with consciousness, the male penis will respond with jerking movements, snaking more deeply into the vagina.

Men can hold the entire penis in awareness, not only the highly magnetic sensitive tip. Feel its full length as it extends marvelously away from the body. Also feel the root of the penis where your penis joins and emerges from the body, and the perineum, the small knotty area between the penis and the rectum. This is the epicenter of the male positive pole, so a man should continually keep the root of the penis in the forefront of his awareness. Don't focus on *where* it is (it can provoke excitement), but *how* it feels; this increases the internal awareness of the penis. Stay connected with this and experience or imagine the penis to be a rod or a magic wand. The greater the consciousness residing in the penis, the more you will be able to rely on its intelligence. The penis will tell you how to make love, when to be still, when to move, and how much to move, in direct response to the environment within the vagina.

The truth is that most men rarely feel the full length of the penis because the interest is on the sensation being created in the tip, usually through repeated rapid movements. But when they do, they have found it to bring an immediately expanded quality to the sexual energy, the feeling of oneself through the penis with power emerging from the root, transmitted along the base upward, and increasing the sensitivity of the head, its magnetic properties. This is advantageous for both men and women as the more sensitive the penis head, the more the delicate and ecstatic vibrations within the vagina can be experienced. This finer magnetic genital functioning is the gift of Tantra, a deeply fulfilling and healing experience for men and women.

KEY POINTS:

ಳಿ Inner focus, slower movements, feeling the genitals from within brings consciousness to them.

ಳಿ Relaxing the pelvic floor repeatedly allows the sexual energy to configure and expand.

- Conscious genitals are tremendously sensitive and alive to each other.

- This is a shift from the "doing" in sex, to the dimension of "being" in sex.

1 0

TOUCH

IMAGINE THE BODY AS A LARGE delectable fruit with soft and juicy parts all over it. You know them, you have felt them in your own body. But how do you touch and stay conscious so that it brings ultimate pleasure to you and your lover? Stroking and caressing your lover as often as possible gives you the chance to experiment with the erotic effects of touch. Notice the subtle responses to your touch and be guided by that. Touch lovingly with awareness in your hands. As you are being touched, close your eyes and allow yourself to *receive* the touch. Absorb the warmth into your own body. Touch and be touched as you make love, it helps enormously to increase sensuality and create sexual presence.

I have found that any type of massage between lovers is an excellent way to begin making love. When massage is done with love and awareness, it quickly creates relaxation, the dropping of tensions, and induces closeness and rapport. Massaging the legs and buttocks has the effect of awakening the sexual energy, especially in women, who tend to hold unexpressed sexual energy in the upper legs, thighs and buttocks. Sometimes this unexpressed sexual energy is reflected in the physical structure, leading to extreme heaviness in the thighs. As consciousness is brought to lovemaking, being touched internally and externally, the body can undergo great changes, replacing imbalance and congestion with balance and fluidity. As the sex energy spreads upward to the heart, slowly we become unified into one graceful whole.

The question is, how to touch and where? The body is full of delectable touchable spots and anywhere is a good place to touch, provided you partner agrees. We all know our bodies and the location of the most sexually sensitive areas, but I suggest that you do not restrict your caresses to such places; it is better to approach them indirectly. Start with a peripheral body part, perhaps the feet, the arms and hands, the head, slowly circling inward and softly toward the back, buttocks, and belly and more sensitive areas. This creates trust and intimacy and the slowness of the approach creates a sensuality and fresh consciousness within the bodies. You will notice your lover's body respond positively in appreciation. Fire grows slowly but surely, and it needs encouragement. It is most likely that your body will be responding in the same way too. Through touch there arises a bodily willingness to make love together, and this changes everything.

Often as we touch one another, we will repeat the same movement or caress again and again. Rubbing up and down, or round and round automatically, almost unaware that we are in fact, touching the body. This lack of consciousness in the touch can unfortunately have an irritating effect on the receiver. She easily feels the lack of consciousness in the hand where there is no tactile communication and so, without sincerity and sensitivity, there is little pleasure in it. While your intention may be to turn your lover on, she may be turning off instead. We can all avoid this by staying aware and conscious while touching.

Communicating through touch

Feel the graceful contours of the body, the supple skin, the silky hair, the bony protrusions. While you are touching, don't focus so much on the *doing*, like stroking or rubbing, but more on feeling of the contact between your hand and their body. Allow your awareness to enter your hand. Relax into *being* and imagine your hand melting or dissolving into their body. The focus on the touch of the hand itself, rather than the activity or the doing, changes the whole quality of the touch. It is quite remarkable. It gives your partner time to feel you, absorb your touch into their body. You will find that your partner warms up and responds much more quickly if your touch is conscious. Feel yourself feeling them, and they feel it too. The sacrum, for example, is always a good place to touch. It feels luscious! With a warm open hand send your love into the base of the spine. It is a sacred place. Feather-light strokes up the spine expand the body energy tremendously. Wrapping the full, open hand around the back of the neck lightly is extremely comforting and reassuring, and this gentle touch can also assist in the release of tears. Or try placing both hands directly over each of the sitz bones, the buttock bones on which we sit. Cup them fully, and to the one receiving, this warmth feels very sexy. Take time to hunt and find special places, juicy spots, and discover how your lover responds. Use your hands to communicate and share your love.

As you touch your lover with awareness, imagine that you are channeling love and warmth into their body. This imagination helps you to get the feeling of energy passing from you into them, and increases communication. Keep your hands in one place for a while, be happy to enjoy the simple touch. Don't do, "be." This kind of conscious touching, without the intention to excite or stimulate your partner, helps them to turn their focus inward to experience themselves. It increases receptivity and sensitivity. For instance, men can be assured that taking fifteen or twenty minutes to lovingly massage their partner's breasts or legs before entering her pays great dividends. It will lead you *both* to greater heights of pleasure and ecstasy. Through serving a woman, a man is fulfilled as a man.

Touching the heart through the breasts

Remembering our background Love Key, Polarity, it is really important that the breasts of a woman be touched before and during lovemaking. Her positive pole needs to be awakened before the negative pole, the vagina, responds with sexual interest. When the female focus is on the clitoris or vagina, and the breasts are ignored, the sexual experience is more likely to be limited to a more linear genital one. When the positive pole, the breasts and heart of woman, is actively engaged, the sexual act takes on a different characteristic. It becomes circular and spontaneous as a deep movement of sexual energy becomes possible.

While making love, most women yearn to have their breasts touched with love and understanding. They intuitively know that it is the breasts that access the deeper layers of sexual energy. When I started being more conscious of the role of the breasts during sex, I found that much to my surprise, they were not very receptive. My relationship with them had always been from the outside, and how they looked as objects, rather than from any inner sense or consciousness of them as breasts. This made them insensitive and unable to absorb the warmth of loving touch. I found that if the breasts and especially the nipples were touched too vigorously or aggressively, it would have the effect of turning me off and causing my body to withdraw, making me less willing to make love. On the other hand, when they were touched in a deliberate or more conscious way without the intention to stimulate, the touch would send sparkles into my vagina. I opened up there and then! Later, when everything was rolling, there would often come a moment when my breasts would be asking for a stronger squeeze or touch and that would continue to open my sexual energy.

I have talked to many women who previously enjoyed having their breasts stimulated when young, then reached a point where they no longer liked to have them touched. They were swollen, congested or over-sensitive, and the nipples very reactive. What can happen is that the breasts, and so the woman as well, become repelled by insensitive touch done without empathy. Frequently, when a man touches a woman's breasts, he is operating from his own desire and enthusiasm and not relating to the breasts themselves. He is touching them in a way that is good for him, but not for her sexual response. A vigorous touch might be more appropriate at some time later during lovemaking, but in the beginning, be deliberate and sensitive. Intend to touch your partner, and then touch with intention. It makes all the difference.

Let your desire, appreciation, love of your partner's breasts be channeled through your hands. Breasts, the symbol of fertility, are indeed beautiful and have captured the eyes and hearts of the artist and the lover for all of humanity. Take the whole breast into the palm of your hand, sending energy and love. Don't do anything for a while, simply "be" with the breast in your hand, perhaps offering a gentle squeeze now and then. Later touch or suck the nipples gently, in a childlike way. Respond to the energy of the breasts and sense how they would like to be touched, not how you would like to touch them. Release your habitual way of reacting to the breasts and nipples, perhaps even your conditioned response to breasts. Caress them with the idea of reaching into your partner, opening her heart in preparation for love. Enter the moment through the presence of your hand.

Caressing the penis

Likewise, a woman should take the penis into her hand and hold it lovingly, embrace it with her hand as if it were a young resilient bird. Again, there is nothing to do with it. Just be with it, feel and absorb its marvelous energy, its strength, its softness. Caress gently and take the testicles into your hands, lightly squeezing them as if they were the most delicate of eggs. Gently massage the testicles between the thumb and forefinger, softly pulling them away from the body. The foreskin and extra folds of skin can be slowly pulled back and away from the head of the penis, exposing the length of the shaft. It feels very good, as well as helping to bring the man's awareness into his penis. The man can focus his awareness, in particular at the root of his penis, his positive pole. Using your hands to communicate in this way with the root of a man will have the effect of creating a vibrant relaxation in his body. In contrast, a stimulating touch to get him hard will place the focus on the excitement aspect of sex, which urges "doing" or orgasm.

Energizing the positive poles of love

Whichever part of the body you are touching, "be" in your hands and send energy through them. A loving, firm and sensitive squeeze is great whenever it feels to be the right moment. As a way to begin making love, mutual touch of the positive poles can be used with great results. The sensitive touch will enable your lover to focus on his penis or her breasts, which awakens the sexual energy without stimulation. This can be done lying on your sides facing each other, or with the man kneeling at the side of the woman who is lying down. Reach out to your partner, and place your relaxed hands on their positive pole. Channel your love and warmth through your hands into them while allowing the eyes to meet. Remain in this mutual exchange for ten to fifteen minutes before you begin making love. It can be difficult to find a position for yourselves where you can be both comfortable and able to touch each other at the same time. If so, one of you touch and the other receive. Then exchange. And then make love.

Remember, this focus on the positive poles of love is very important as it sets the stage for the interplay of polarity once penetration occurs. When the opposite poles are alive to each other, the penis and vagina in attunement, an incredible interchange of energy is possible. Lovemaking can become increasingly dynamic, the bodies twisting and turning around and into each other for hours, as if possessed by life itself.

Remember it is very helpful to communicate to your lover what you are feeling in your body as you are being touched. Use a few simple words; begin a conscious dialogue between you and your body to intensify your awareness. Share your now!

When considering touch, don't limit yourself to the idea of hands only. Be aware of the bodies themselves touching each other, where they touch, how they touch, and the silky slippery feelings between legs, arms, lips, bellies, chests. While embracing and kissing, be alert initially not to push your bodies hard up against each other in too much enthusiasm! This has the unfortunate affect of compressing the physical body and with it the energy field surrounding the body, which limits or eradicates all sensuous feelings. There will be a lack of porousness, and consciousness will not be able to filter through the body. They will be perceived as solid unyielding objects which limits receptivity.

You have most likely felt this difference when you have a hug with someone. One person may give you a hug or handshake, squeezing you a little too hard, or even slapping you on the back taking your breath away, without any real exchange of energy or warmth. Another person may surprise you by simply melting into your arms. Suddenly you feel vaporous and light, expanded through the contact. A touching sweetness arises out of the simplicity.

As is the way of Tantra, touch begins with you and a slow sensitive approach in order for energy and aliveness to flourish in the cells of the body. Take the time to sense yourself as you lie down. Breathe for a few minutes, turn to your lover and face him. Feel the space between you that separates and connects you. Allow the eyes to meet and move the bodies together inch by inch. More subtle phenomena need time and tranquillity in which to grow, and this creates an environment conducive to energy and electricity within the body. When the touch of your bodies is sensitive, porous, and conscious, the relaxed sexual energy can become a spontaneous and dynamic force.

KEY POINTS:

ৡ Touching, stroking and caressing is a natural expression of love.

ৡ Use relaxed friendly hands, conscious and slow, molding to the body curves and shapes.

ৡ Channel energy and warmth through the hands to access the female sexual energy through the breasts.

క్రReceive the warmth radiating from a loving hand, accept and absorb the touch into your body.

I I

RELAXATION

THROUGH ACTIVITY AND EFFORT and tension, we achieve our aims, fulfill our plans and projects. Through relaxation we achieve a more loving heart and a greater sense of well-being. Most of us are longing for the state of relaxation where we experience deep inner peace, each moment a joy, without disturbing and anxious thoughts about the future. As we experiment with the Love Keys we are learning to relax in many different ways, to enable a more loving and nourishing exchange to arise through sex. When we remove the idea that we must get something out of sex, we find we can begin to relax. No longer is an orgasm the all-important goal that has to be reached through effort and tension every time. When it happens it is good, and when it does not happen it is also good.

There arises an acceptance of what is, because there is no pressure of what should be. This acceptance leads to realizing and appreciating what is actually happening, the delightful joys within the body, the simple breath, the feelings that come and go, the alertness that arises with an inward focus—all this creates a deep sexual relaxation. In this frame of mind we are able to welcome whatever comes next, almost cat-like, self-contained and purring, while completely responsive to our changing environment. We have all envied cats their tranquillity while admiring their impeccable alertness. We must bring relaxation into the sexual act so that it becomes a magical unfolding rather than a fixed routine. We must become children again, utterly absorbed in the seashells littering the glistening shore. Sooner or later in life many of us, whether consciously or unconsciously, find ourselves searching in different ways to regain this lost childhood absorption and peace.

The power of doing less and being more

The state of exhaustion or laziness where you are uninvolved, detached and bored or groggy and sleepy, is often described as one of relaxation, but it isn't. Relaxation returns you to earth rejuvenated, not devastated. Relaxation is the process of becoming increasingly alive. It is a powerful force. If you have ever had the heart-warming experience of your finger being encircled with gripping life force by a tiny baby, this demonstrates the power of relaxation from a child without muscular strength. True relaxation happens when you pull your attention from without to within, external to internal, from activity to rest, doing less and being more. If, when you lie down to rest in the afternoon, you slowly and consciously bring different parts of the body into the awareness through relaxation, and then remain in that awareness for fifteen or twenty minutes, you will notice the refreshing results it produces. Relaxation regenerates the body and uplifts the spirit. You emerge as a different person. Importantly, relaxation is not a collapse of the physical structure as many people believe, but a returning of presence to the physical structure. When you relax consciously, you enter the body parts, become more alert, more vibrant, more sensitive and receptive. It is not a checking out but more a checking in. So while making love, you do not disappear and leave your partner, instead you arrive in your body, poised and present to your partner.

Tension, the opposite of relaxation, reflects itself in the body as hardness of muscles and body tissues. Having touched countless bodies in therapeutic massage clinics over many years, I have found the upper back, shoulder and neck area of most people to feel like concrete, solid and thick, creating a feeling of immense density. The cells of the body are compressed through internal and external pressures, and there is simply not enough space for physical comfort. Too many people report tiredness and anxiety, neck pain, headaches, eyestrain, difficulties in breathing and sleeping. When we do not feel physically well it affects our psychological state considerably, and can easily determine our happiness or unhappiness. Physical therapies are an answer as these encourage physical and mental relaxation, but one hour of massage or exercise will not correct years of accumulated tension. Relaxation is an ongoing deepening process that never really ends. The body is composed of 70 to 80 percent water, like a huge elastic bag, jelly-like, but most of our bodies have lost this soft and watery quality. Through consciousness and relaxation the body is able to revert to its smooth, soft state.

Perhaps the most difficult aspect of relaxation is convincing ourselves that it is something of genuine merit. Is it really beneficial to do so? How many times did you think about lying down to rest, but your mind soon convinced you otherwise, saying "I must *do* something?" So you performed a long-awaited task, for which you could later congratulate yourself. And yet, if you had spent the morning relaxing comfortably in bed, you might have felt guilty thinking it was time wasted, or misspent. Relaxation is given no intrinsic value in our lives. This same compulsion to do something is found even more forcefully in sex.

Giving up control for expansion

So, in our new approach to lovemaking, we have to introduce relaxation by reducing the amount of physical effort we make. It implies relaxing the body and its movements (slowing down to achieve genital consciousness), and it also implies relaxing the mind. At this point it is often hard to believe that forgetting about orgasm and choosing to relax instead is going to be worthwhile! Our minds, our sexual conditioning, our past experiences, will urgently talk us out of relaxing, by saying "Go for it, it's so nice anyway, what could be better?" In effect, by relaxing, we are releasing our control over the sexual act, and the aspects of our sexual expression that keeps us locked into habits. It is not so easy for the mind to accept the idea of less control, so reason will be determined to keep you contracted and within your normal range of experience. However, when we do manage to relax underneath the urge for orgasm or "doing," we will find the experience full of richness and variety. It astounds me how many layers of relaxation are possible. Just when I sense my body or mind is fully relaxed, I find yet an additional layer of subtle tension. With each drop into relaxation, there is a corresponding sense of expansion within the body, awareness of more subtle vibrations. There arises a sense of glowing and porous life at an intercellular level.

As you make love, travel around your body again and again to find any areas of tension, the places where you are unconsciously contracting your muscles. It could be the shoulders, the inner thighs, the feet, the belly, the jaw, the anus. Anywhere. Each drop in relaxation counts. Tightness in the jaw is often related to tension in the pelvic area, so again and again bring your awareness to the jaw and relax it as you make love. It is well worth it. As you play around with relaxing different parts of the body in this way, you will notice how the smallest of tensions affect your sexual energy. As you release them, even if there appears to be no direct relationship between the body parts, for instance the shoulders and the penis or the feet and the vagina, you will feel an increase in sexual sensations.

Not unlike the pelvic floor, the solar plexus too is a place to relax and instill with consciousness, especially as you make love. Here too, we gather and store many unconscious tensions including the debilitating effects of painful emotional experiences. It is therefore not an area in which we have much consciousness. However, when the solar plexus is relaxed and filled with awareness, the sexual exchange between man and woman changes. It brings genuine spontaneity into the sex act, and enables you to hold the awareness within while being fully responsive to the outer events. This area may not be easy to sense initially, or it may bring feelings of nausea or a lump in the stomach, a sure sign of fears and tensions stored in the body. In time these negative feelings are released. Once it is easier to access this area, it is a suggestion to lovers that they hold their awareness in the solar plexus as they make love. The fire of awareness built up here spills warmth over into the genitals. When we are present, we are truly passionate. This engagement with the solar plexus has the capacity to squeeze out the tiring thoughts through which we always filter our experience. There is a strong sensation of being fully within and without simultaneously. Men happily report that the urge to ejaculate diminishes, and there is an ease and relaxation from which a power emerges.

Relaxing into sexual energy

The response to relaxation is innate; we are born with it. I sometimes call it the sixth sense. If one person is fully relaxed and present the other person will automatically be affected and become more relaxed and present themselves. For instance, when a woman relaxes deeply in lovemaking, without actually doing anything but focusing on receiving and being present instead, automatically her partner will become more conscious, sensitive, and loving. He will naturally align with the present, and thoughts of orgasm will not even arise. Instead a magical doorway opens and the man perceives something completely different happening to him. It is an unforgettable experience. For the first time he has been able to make love without effort or tension. It is more of a dance, a sensuous winding of bodies. So never feel that you must wait for the other to relax before you can; relaxation starts with you first and foremost.

Accumulated tensions held in the body have an exhausting effect on it, so when couples change the way they make love, and begin to relax, they often report feeling very tired, real sleepiness, the desire to collapse or an actual physical weakness in the muscles. Perhaps they even experience low blood pressure. This is a sure sign that relaxation is beginning. The old tensions are surfacing through the tiredness, and it is not a cause for alarm. The chronic unfelt fatigue surfaces acutely, and in this way is released from the body. It is very beneficial. Take plenty of rest, and do not be in a hurry to go somewhere or do something. When relaxation in sex is achieved, it is the closest you can actively get to the foundation of your energy system. Relaxation here at the source will have a ripple effect on every level: mind, body, and spirit. The benefits are almost immediate without having to do more or less than make love.

In essence, when we are no longer hooked or driven by our sexual desires, when mind and body can truly relax into the present moment and its glory, we experience the backflow of our own sexual energy. Instead of forcing it to a release, we relax and allow the energy to languidly fall back on itself, and then rise inward and upward. In this way relaxation is essential to Tantra. It requires an unhurried and timeless approach; if you have made love for three or four hours or more, you will know the deep sense of peace and love it brings. This rare quality radiates from within you.

An effortless surrender

Time is only important when we have an objective to fulfill, somewhere to go. Without such aims, there is absolutely no need to hurry. You can relax and take a long, slow walk, enjoying sensual delights and so lift sex to a new frequency. Through this relaxation the sexual energy is reabsorbed by the body. Set aside a few hours so that you do not have to think about the time because time always brings tension. Through this, relaxation will be easier. Be playful, touch, caress, kiss. Take time to know each other physically and allow an attunement to arise between the bodies, let it be a slow, gradual coming together. What we are trying to create within our bodies is a tranquil environment, not an excited one. It's an important step if you wish to experiment with sex as an uplifting force. It is the difference between pleasure and ecstasy! Through making the initial effort of *not* making an effort in sex, a kind of ease emerges, a surrendering to the life force as it begins to move through the bodies with magnetic intelligence, seeking and searching completion through the other. As we relax more and more into sex, we find the refreshing quality of relaxation pervading our lives, making us alert, joyful, loving, and creative.

KEY POINTS:

ဆ Sexual energy functions best in a relaxed environment.

ဆ Use awareness to search for, and relax, unconscious tensions.

ဆ Reduce the amount of physical effort in sex.

ဆ The more you relax, the more the other person relaxes, deepening the experience.

12

SOFT PENETRATION

BECAUSE THE SEXUAL ORGANS are full of the accumulated tension of past experiences, they are no longer able to function according to their true polarity. Having lost their innate sensitivity, the vaginal walls are not found to be in their natural state; moist and slippery like the inside of the oyster. Instead of the texture one feels when eating soft fleshy coconut, they have become toughened and unyielding from years of friction. In the same way, a man's penis, which in its natural state is snake-like, firm and flexible, can become hard and rigid, almost metallic, as it swells, full of energy that cannot be rightly channeled into a woman.

This tension in the genitals, which has affected the male and female polarity, must gradually be dissolved and emptied out so that the original polarities can be restored. The penis must once again become a vehicle for generating and transmitting energy into a woman, while the vagina becomes capable of inviting, absorbing, receiving, and circulating this male energy. As the penis and vagina become more relaxed, freed of their restricting tensions, the positive energy of the male and the negative energy of the female begin to challenge each other, with a pushing and pulling effect, creating a delicate and ecstatic magnetic sexual exchange, far more penetrating than the pleasures of friction-based sex could ever be.

A good way to start restoring polarity is to attempt soft penetration—yes, without an erection! This idea is often greeted with laughter and disbelief, but it is a reality, the penis can go inside when it is not erect and it feels remarkably wonderful. It can be inserted by the woman or the man. Importantly, soft penetration also takes the pressure off the man by disproving the assumption that the penis must be erect in order to make love. Managing to insert the relaxed penis in the vagina is a knack that takes some practice, but it is well worth it. Furthermore, if a man is having difficulties in achieving an erection without stimulation, or if he suffers from impotence, soft penetration means that he can still enter a woman and make love to her.

When the penis is inserted in its relaxed state, the man is given the opportunity to be more present, since the pressure of having to have an erection can often lead to psychological distress or sexual fantasy. With soft penetration this pitfall is eliminated. In conventional sex the man, according to his positive polarity, will usually be ready for sex well before the woman whose sexual temperature is naturally lower. Through soft penetration this difference can be overcome, and the man and woman can warm up together, the genitals slowly greeting and growing into fullness. The penis can become erect *inside* the vagina in direct response to the vaginal environment, which creates an entirely different quality of sexual energy to that of penetration with erection. The genitals have a chance to attune to each other without the pressure of having to make something happen. This lack of pressure to perform begins to restore balance to the penis and vagina; accumulated tensions are emptied out, slowly returning to their naturally responsive state.

Take the time to love consciously

It is possible that in the beginning it may be difficult to feel anything at all in the penis or the vagina, let alone something interesting or pleasurable. Suddenly you are in a gap. Imagine that someone is rubbing your back vigorously for several minutes and they suddenly stop. It wouldn't be so easy to feel the motionless hand at first. It would take a while to sense the energy and warmth spreading from the hand into your back, because it is infinitely more subtle than the heat created through the friction of rubbing. Likewise, if the genitals are accustomed to friction as a way of communicating, the contrast of no movement or less movement will initially produce less feeling. The subtle tingling electrical sensitivity between the penis and vagina during soft penetration is so delicate, it takes some time to grow into the feeling of it. It is certainly worth every moment of waiting though, because after a time the genitals begin to buzz together, and the idea of sex as some kind of doing or an effort begins to change.

A man dedicated to conscious loving commented, "Until I experienced simple soft penetration, the penis did not have any real sense of meaningful direction." He found that when he relaxed consciously while being soft inside the vagina, his penis would gradually become erect, as if drawn up into depths of the vagina with an intelligence of its own. This inherent direction of the penis is an electro-magnetic phenomenon and it is not something you can "do." In fact it is our "*doing*" that prevents it happening. If a couple can relax with soft penetration *(see* fig. 7), and increase their genital awareness and presence, they will

Fig.7   Side position for soft penetration

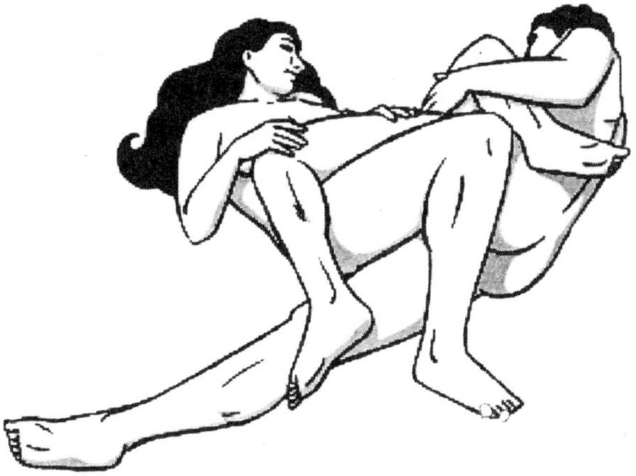

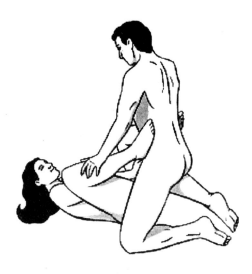

Fig.8   Middle position for soft penetration

start to discover a new level of sexual experience with the penis developing snake-like qualities as it writhes ecstatically into the vagina, sucked inward by the opposing polarity. The more conscious you are as you make love, the more readily the intrinsic polarities will be restored to the genitals.

Positions for soft penetration

The position for soft penetration is easy *(see* fig. 7). The man lies on his side facing the woman. The woman lies on her back, bringing her pelvis close to his. Both open their legs, and the genitals will be naturally lying opposite each other. Bring them together, and wrap your legs around each other. This is sometimes called the scissors position. The woman may have to move her upper body away from her lover's in order to make the pelvises fit, or she can angle her own pelvis upward. Experiment and do what is most comfortable. This does not work for every couple. Lying between the legs of the woman for soft penetration, and rolling onto the sides from time to time, is a good alternative. In this middle position *(see* fig. 8) it is easy for a man to insert the penis.

How the woman inserts the penis

For soft penetration in the side position, once you are positioned correctly, pelvises close together, with vagina opposite penis, the woman can proceed with the soft penetration by taking the penis in her hands (see fig. 9). If you need lubricant, now would be the perfect moment to apply it, but don't make it too slippery to handle. Slowly pull back the folds of foreskin around the head of the penis, and expose it with the skin pulled away and down toward the root. Now make a two-pronged fork with the first two fingers of both hands (short fingernails please!) Place one finger fork (try the left hand) firmly around the base of the penis and hold it there. With the other hand (the right) place the fingers directly either side and behind the rim encircling the head of the penis. Squeeze the fingers together so that you have a gentle grip on the penis, and then pull the penis toward your vagina. When it arrives at the entrance begin to insert it. You will be able to push it in and up a little way. Do the same thing again. Grip the penis between your two fingers, and direct it into your vagina. By repeating the finger movement again and again, it is as if you're feeding or walking the penis into the vagina, gently pushing it inside a

Fig. 9   Finger position for soft penetration

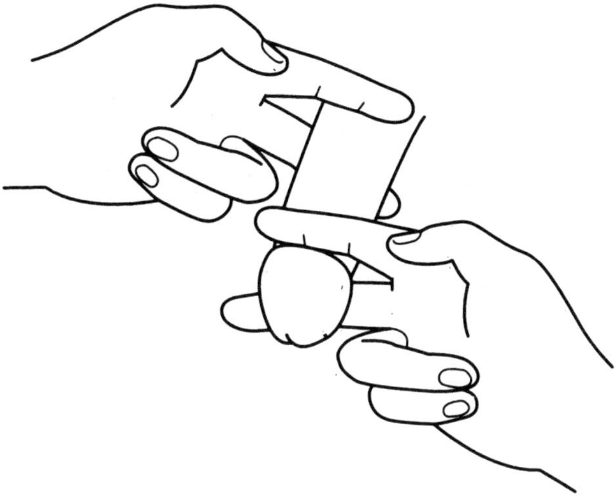

little more each time. Once you have pushed all of it inside you (or as much as you can manage to insert—even to get the head in is a good start), remove your hands, and bring the pelvic areas together as closely as possible, then wrap your legs around each other and relax! Use pillows to make yourselves as comfortable as you can, and use other Love Keys to support your presence. In this position eye contact is easy and important, as is breathing, and it is possible too for the man to rest a hand on the woman's breasts while she can stroke his buttocks and thighs.

You *absolutely must* keep your vagina relaxed during the soft penetration, or it will be like 'trying to force your lover through a closed door. It simply won't work. As you insert the penis, it is most likely that you will want to look between your legs at what you are doing, especially at first. You will do this by lifting your upper body through contracting the belly musculature. When the belly contracts, so does the vagina and to avoid this tightening, send your awareness consciously downward into the vagina in order to keep it relaxed and open. I have found that lying back for a moment, and consciously relaxing my vagina once I have a hold of the penis and before insertion, helps me to widen and relax the vaginal muscles. Once you have done this, slip the soft penis in. As the penis and vagina relax, the easier soft penetration becomes. You can use soft penetration as a way of approaching lovemaking every time if you wish, or use it when you need it. But never forget it.

A new sexual language

As you begin this new experience, it is important to remember to communicate what you are feeling. For instance, when a man hears from his partner that she can feel energy radiating from his soft, yet unerect penis, that is a great relief. Discovering that he is alive when soft is extremely reassuring. He can stop worrying about erection and focus his attention on the direct experience of the penis within the vagina. This is a far more subtle level of perception and requires a quietness of mind and an absence of anxious thoughts.

Bringing the bodies together in this way is limited in excitement and opens up all kinds of other possibilities for sexual exchange. Just leave it up to the genitals supported by your consciousness, and they will do whatever feels right to them. It is a completely new sexual language. The penis may lie in the vagina, humming quietly and contentedly, or after a while it may start vibrating strongly. It may become slowly and steadily erect, pushing high up into the vagina, dancing and jerking upward, or relax down again, snaking all the way out, only to rise back up again in thrilling penetration. Through this meeting of opposites all kinds of miracles happen.

KEY POINTS:

↝ Soft penetration is easy and a wonderful way to start making love.

↝ It means you can warm up together and be relaxed about it.

↝ "Share your now" to increase awareness and genital sensitivity.

↝ An erection can grow in response to the vagina, a thrilling sexual experience.

↝ Sexual energy arises from the interplay of male and female polarities.

13

DEEP PENETRATION

GENERATIONS OF WOMEN have failed to experience their divine orgasmic potential, the female delight of sensuality and love through sex. The Garden of Love, the secret gateway to sexual ecstasy for women and men, lies abandoned, untouched, and overgrown with straying weeds. All the emotional memories of a woman's painful sexual experiences such as rape, abortion, aggression, and abuse leave their psychological imprint in this deepest part of the vagina. This causes constriction in the vaginal tissues, making the walls tough and unyielding. In this way, there is an ongoing protective defense set up in the tissues, and the vagina contracts instinctively during intercourse, inhibiting deeper penetration. This means that the powerful positive penis head is unable to correspond smoothly and directly with its negative counterpart in the very depths of the vagina, thus affecting the energy flow.

Women's sexual ecstasy

For a woman to experience these ecstatic energies in the depths of her vagina, the tensions and disturbance created by past events must slowly be released so that the woman's negative pole becomes simple and innocent with a welcoming receptivity. She is then able to fully receive and utilize the positive male energy to circulate within her. The more sensitized the penis and vagina are to each other, and the longer a couple make love in this trusting way, the more it leads to an ecstatic experience of lovemaking. The energy exchange between the sexual organs is thrilling enough to root you firmly in the here and now, creating the dimension of Tantra very naturally.

Penetrate the depths and stay still

To strengthen the original nature of this polarity effect in our organs of love, they need to be consciously healed and purified of toxic tensions. This is done through deep, sustained penetration. For the woman, the focal area for healing is located deep at the top of the vagina. It includes the sides of the upper vaginal canal and up and around the cervix, which protrudes into this part of the vagina. This is her Garden of Love, the place where she will first know true ecstasy in sex. When a woman is touched this deeply and consciously by the penis, she may experience real love in her body through sex for the first time. A friend experienced it as a pearl rolling all the way up from the penis into her heart. Here where she is pure woman, her heart opens beautifully and naturally, but it so rarely happens. Instead, penetration is limited to short thrusts focused on the first few centimeters of the vagina where several strong rings of muscle are found encircling the entrance. Friction-like rapid movements back and forth at the entrance have the effect of creating intense pleasure, which leads to excitement and thereby an interest in orgasm. Through this, women's interest has been drawn away from the awareness of this jewel in her upper vagina. Seldom has she had the opportunity to feel it with true tenderness, and thus the source of her true femininity lies untapped.

Women (and men's) dependence on the clitoris for female orgasm has not helped matters as far as vaginal consciousness is concerned. Countless women do not know the satisfaction of a full vaginal orgasm, and so for many of us the clitoris becomes the prime focus while making love. By making aggressive thrusting pelvic movements aimed at stimulating the clitoris, she is able to create the necessary excitement for orgasm. Men too have become accustomed to giving women sexual satisfaction through the clitoris. The outcome of a lot of sexual excitement has been a relative desensitizing of the vagina. In the upper part she is protective, and in the lower part she is tense, tough, and expectant.

Restoring masculine and feminine polarities

In its unequaled wisdom, nature gives us the perfect instrument to rectify the situation. This power is found in the potency of the penis. Deep, sustained penetration by the penis, in fact, is the best way to restore both the masculine and feminine polarities. Incredibly, the head of the penis acts like a highly sensitive magnet entering the energy field of the feminine pole. This has a dramatic effect on the accumulated vaginal tensions, precipitating a discharge or dispersal experienced in a number of ways, and in time the area is gradually transformed so as to generate exquisite feminine energies. Through this both poles are strengthened. As an integral part of this healing process in the vagina, the sensitivity and flexibility and consciousness will also be returned to the penis itself. Men too, have accumulated tensions and pains through misunderstanding, misuse, and abuse of their wonderful male antennae. This disturbance has led to two predominant male extremes, one where there is too much tension in sex leading to premature ejaculation, and the other is impotence, a lack of response or sensitivity in the penis due to sexual atrophy. Both these imbalances can be restored by removing the tensions accumulated in the male genitals.

Deep penetration is the way to contact the divine energies of woman and for man to experience his true sexual potency. When a woman's body is lovingly prepared, her heart incorporated, she becomes utterly sensual, and will respond spontaneously to love, which is deeply satisfying to a man. Here lies his true male authority, to be selfless enough to fully love a woman and give to her. The woman feels that her life has been enriched energetically by being able to receive active energy, and the man becomes receptive by being able to give, creating a circle in this exchange that fills us with the radiance of love.

Deep *sustained* penetration should be approached as a *style* of lovemaking, rather than something you do occasionally. Do so whenever it is possible. A full erection is required and if the man finds that he is not fully erect, he can use a little movement but he must avoid too much excitement. There should be just enough movement or arousal for a soft, supple erection, not more. If the state of erection arises from soft penetration, then slowly move into the depths of the vagina. To do this you can

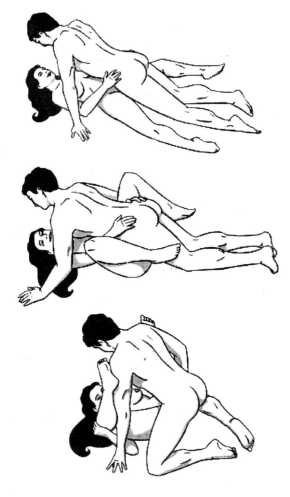

Fig.10   Positions for deep sustained penetration

artfully change position by shifting limbs around, if possible without the penis losing contact with the vagina, so that the man is then kneeling between the woman's legs. She pulls her legs up to her chest, and curls the pelvis upward to deepen or change the angle of the penetration. Use some of the other Love Keys at the same time too, such as eyes meeting, breathing deeply and slowly, communication, and awareness in the genitals (see fig. 10).

Slow and porous approach

Any heavy thrust or insensitive approach will cause the woman to tighten her vagina in automatic defense, so penetrate consciously as slowly as possible, millimeter by millimeter. Go in as far as you can or until you feel some resistance against the head of your penis. You may be touching the cervix, the opening to the uterus, or the sides and upper boundaries of the vaginal canal. Once you have arrived there, keep the penis still. Don't move. Hold your awareness and attention in the head of the penis, feeling from the root upward. Do not push up hard against the vaginal tissues; this is important. Once you feel you have gone as deep as possible into the vagina, simply pull back a hair's breadth. Really as little as that! It makes all the difference, and will not affect your pleasure in any way. Surprisingly, you are likely to feel more and not less. Allow the contact between the penis and vagina to be "porous", light and airy. If you push up hard you will compact the cells of the vagina, which will defend against your intrusion, pushing you away rather than receiving you. A tiny bit of porous space enables the male and female energy to mingle, allowing the dispersing effect to take place. When this fraction of space is not given, the feeling is one of being flattened up against a wall.

After a time of continued contact a pulsation or throbbing may begin in the head of the penis at the point where it is touching the vaginal walls. When you feel this, remain still and present for as long as you can, relaxing into the changing sensations. Be with whatever is. It is good, over time, to open the vagina up from all angles; there is more space up and around the cervix than we appreciate. To encourage exploration of the untouched upper aspects of the vagina, the man should move his pelvis (and thus the penis) *slowly* to the side, to the right or to the left, and then hold still. This is not to be mistaken for a back and forth movement, rather it is a shift to the side whereby the man is changing the angle of his pelvis, which then enables the penis to reach more remote areas. Then wait, allowing the intelligence of the penis to guide you. It may begin to move of its own accord, seeking out areas of hidden tensions, or be delightfully sucked upward by the vagina. This magnetic intelligence is profoundly touching, a union of man and woman, body and heart.

The woman should remain still and receptive, focusing on her breasts and relaxing her vagina, holding the awareness deep inside where the penis is making contact. It will feel ecstatic, a heightened sensitivity, sometimes almost overwhelming, as a completely different sexual experience arises. At the outset the man may feel a shooting, buzzing, or electrical energy in his penis or through his body and he must stay here and now with this intense feeling of pleasure. It is a tremendous thrill, and the woman will also feel corresponding sensations, sometimes like relaxed waves of orgasm. Or the whole area begins to glow golden, steadily increasing in intensity, spreading throughout the body. As you make love, keep exploring new positions which deepen penetration. To enhance this exchange, imagine your organs to be generators of love energy.

It may happen that after a time of this ecstatic exchange, the penis unexpectedly begins to withdraw and the man will begin to lose his erection. This can be very alarming, but it is a process of nature, action, and rest. Once the penis has transformed some energies it naturally subsides into a relaxed state. If a couple can continue to keep their consciousness in the penis and vagina as this happens, and remain still rather than move or lose interest, the penis will usually rise up again into the depths of the vagina.

Healing sexual pain and memories

At first, it is possible that this deliberate contact through the sustained deep penetration may feel sharp or painful in some places, and a woman might have the impulse to move away. It can also feel a bit numb or distant, even deadened. It is good to understand that the pain or numbness is usually reflecting some sort of tension or cellular memory held in the tissue. Some women have felt a pain reflecting to the anus or the lower back, down the legs and to areas where there may already be other physical troubles. The amount of pain, tension, and emotion present in a woman's vagina is directly related to her personal sexual history. Whatever degree of pain or abuse we may have suffered, we all have our individual sexual past and its agonies sitting directly over our feminine pole. These pains and memories are often unconscious, and we are rarely aware of them. But when we slow down and bring consciousness to healing the genitals, old emotional pains buried in the past may surface. The first sign of pain or discomfort is not to be avoided. Pain is an invitation, an indication of tension; pain indicates that healing touch is needed. It is important that the woman does not allow her man to push strongly into this pain. We are definitely not interested in adding pain to pain; so let him in only as deeply as feels comfortable to you. Communicate to him what is happening to you. Rather than pushing him out, ask him to move back a little, even a hair's breadth can be enough. Breathe, be interested, relax and allow the penis to transform the pain.

Often the pain will turn to intense pleasure or tears. This is a release of buried emotional tension, which has created hardness, and lack of vaginal receptivity. The tears, the pain, coughing, and any laughter that may arise seemingly out of the blue are all signs that the vagina is softening and relaxing. If you are lucky enough to experience this kind of release, you will notice an immediate (and I mean immediate) change in the sensitivity of your vagina. Suddenly your perception is heightened as the joy and vitality of life spreads into the area. The man too, will feel a profound expansion, an intensification of pleasure and greater sensitivity in his penis.

In the same way, a man can also experience a spontaneous release of emotions, feel shooting pains, burning sensations, grateful tears of relief, and with it an immediate strengthening of his authentic male energy. Where pain persists after the lovemaking it can signify an unexpressed emotional component, so a man is encouraged to allow himself to express his hidden feelings. Using sound to express the pain, finding a sound that vibrates from within the pain itself, and anything that flows from that expression, is one way to release these tensions.

With this dissolving of tensions through the sustained conscious presence of the penis in the vagina, a healing process is set in motion. The penis heals and transforms the vagina, and in so doing, the penis itself is healed and transformed. It arises as a consequence of its transforming power, and an innate circle is completed, penis and vagina are healed through each other; natural balance is restored to man and woman. For such reasons, Tantra is described as a process of great purification. We release the past by purifying ourselves of its tensions, which restrict the sexual energy and its glorious expansion. As the genitals become more pure, simple, and innocent, they are able to generate sexual energy and this transforms the act. It becomes quiet, still, and serene. As the innate magnetic intelligence is returned to the sexual organs, it becomes a moving spiritual force, a joyful inspiration. At last we are able to touch and be touched by the other.

KEY POINTS:

৪→ Male "positive" and female "negative" generate ecstatic streaming energies.

৪→ Women's divine feminine energies are located in the upper part of the vagina.

৪→ This ecstatic "Garden of Love" is to be consciously awakened by deep, sustained "porous" penetration.

।❛∝The head of the penis is similar to a powerful magnet.

❛∝As the consciousness in the penis and vagina is purified, sexual ecstasy increases.

❛∝Let sustained penetration be a "style" of lovemaking whenever erection is present.

I4

ROTATING POSITIONS

IN TANTRIC SEX, position itself is not important; who is in the position is what matters. Therefore there are no specially prescribed positions for Tantra because it is the people who make the positions. The idea is that you make the position work. If you are present, breathing, and relaxed, almost any position will be the right one for you, but you must be fully within yourself to create a new sexual reality. This is the sexual present of Tantra, the awareness of life within the body.

Genital communion

The most significant thing about any position is that it should enhance genital communion, adding depth and contact between the penis and vagina. And it should be comfortable. Otherwise when there is strain in the body the awareness becomes distracted. The position you choose should enhance the sensitivity and the experience—which may be a tingling or streaming or a feeling of electrical exchange or whatever else is present. With our new understanding of the penis and vagina as complementary poles, two parts of one unit, we can now transform our general thinking about positions and movement in sex. It is highly advantageous if they fit snugly into each other, so as to increase the energetic potential. It is wonderful too, when a woman spreads her labia open after (or before) penetration as this makes the contact more sensual. Penetrate as deeply as you can and at the same time let it be a "porous" contact, remembering that pushing unduly hard against the vaginal walls will negate this magnetic sensitivity. In Tantra, whichever position you are in, the idea is to allow the bodies to remain together or move as a single unit, keeping the penis and vagina as an unmoving focal point. When we keep this in mind, the bodies themselves find creative positions around the genital connection.

The thrusting pelvic movements in regular sex are generally done in opposition to each other; you pull away from and then push towards each other at the same time. Backwards and forwards you move, forcing the penis in and out of the vagina without any time for real correspondence between them. But in Tantra, when you move as a unit, the penis does not leave the vagina. It stays all the way within the depths of the vagina, and the bodies rotate and move around this primary connection (see fig. 11), each position contributing to the sexual exchange. The thrill of these rotating shifts in position easily replaces the pattern of thrusting and friction-like movements in sex. Men will also find some succulent movement is possible within the vagina without actually moving out or creating any friction, and this is delightful. As a man grows in sensitivity and stillness, his penis will begin to direct him in how to make love, letting him know when to shift position or move, and when to be probing or still. This authority and trust given by the man to his penis changes the lovemaking into a divine experience.

Experimenting with rotating positions, keeping your awareness

Since sexual energy is a dynamic living force, not at all static, it will keep on changing and moving. Therefore you must be alert, shifting and changing the bodies according to what is happening between the genitals. Rotate around the genital connection, and you will find that an interesting sequence of rotating positions is possible if you start, for instance, in the scissors position described for soft penetration.

Without being too inventive, any number of positions can

easily be found. In fact with every centimeter you move, your bodies configure into a new position. Take time to experiment with it and see how easily the bodies can roll around together! To begin with, you can explore possibilities *without* penetration. Lie on a carpeted floor together in any position and imagine the genitals are joined. Then, keeping the pelvises glued together, (so the penis does not leave the vagina), start to change position by moving the bodies in unison, and you will find a sequence of positions emerging. Hold each position for a few minutes and then shift again. With this flexibility and

Fig. 11   Sequence of rotating positions through front

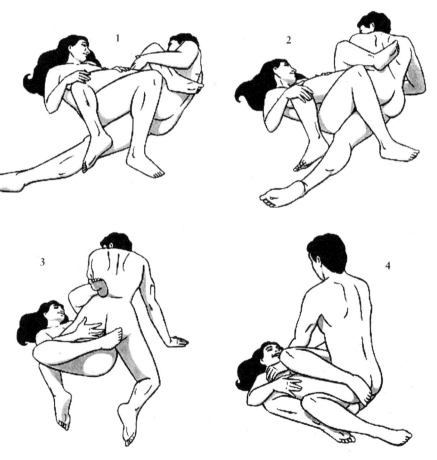

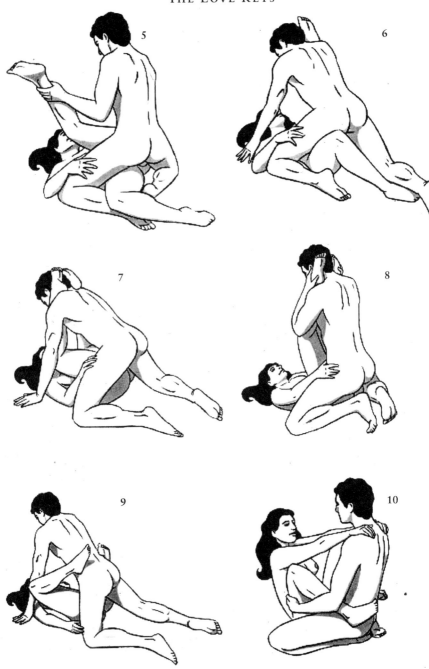

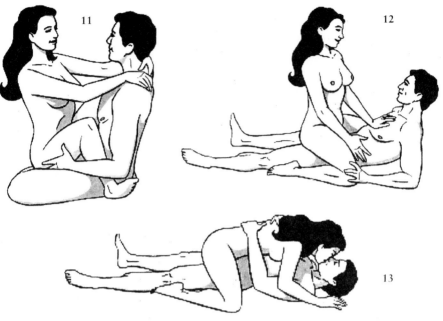

choice the body can find the right position for the moment, whether the moment is a second or an hour. When you keep the attention on this connection between poles and the energy exchange, you can support it with the bodies. When the two bodies are well proportioned, they can become one fluid ball of energy rolling around with its own momentum.

Changing position creates presence

When you focus on awareness and presence, the position of the mind is more important than that of the body. If you change your mind you may then want to change your positions. So with this new understanding, begin to trust and appreciate the wisdom of your body and give way to it. When the body has a spontaneous impulse, allow it rather than listen to the mind. If you suddenly have the urge to turn over and make love on top, but an inner voice reminds you of times when you did that and he lost his erection, try it anyway. Drop the voices of the past and yield to the present. Be as alive to yourself as you can. When the body chooses a position that makes you feel vulnerable and exposed, it means you are "here," it is something new, unknown. Stay in this position for some time. Don't move out of it to release your discomfort, but remember instead that this is the intensity of the present moment. In the same way, if you find yourself drifting away into thought, or you feel sleepy and absent, change your position. This immediately brings a change in the genital connection and helps you to regain presence.

Once you begin to understand how sexual energy best responds, you will find that at least initially, old favored positions no longer support you in your new orientation. For example, when the man is on top he will most likely feel an incredible pressure to do something, because in the past he has always thrust his pelvis from this position. At first it can be difficult to "be" in a position, while your body and mind are longing to "do" something. To enable the man to relax more easily, the woman can assume the superior position. When I first tried this, as soon as I was on top I felt as if I had to do something too, I could easily feel awkward and unnatural, or pressured, and it took some time to relax into "being." But I have also learned that when I am in a true sexual flow, my body and that of my lover will simply take the position that is needed.

With this in mind, there are a variety of positions that two bodies can create, so be imaginative and keep changing *(see* fig. 12). You don't have to disconnect to do so, but remember to *rotate* around the genitals, and if the penis slips out of the

Fig. 12   Sequence of rotating positions through rear

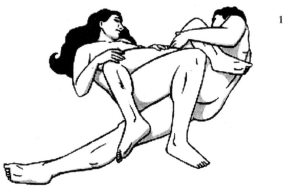

1

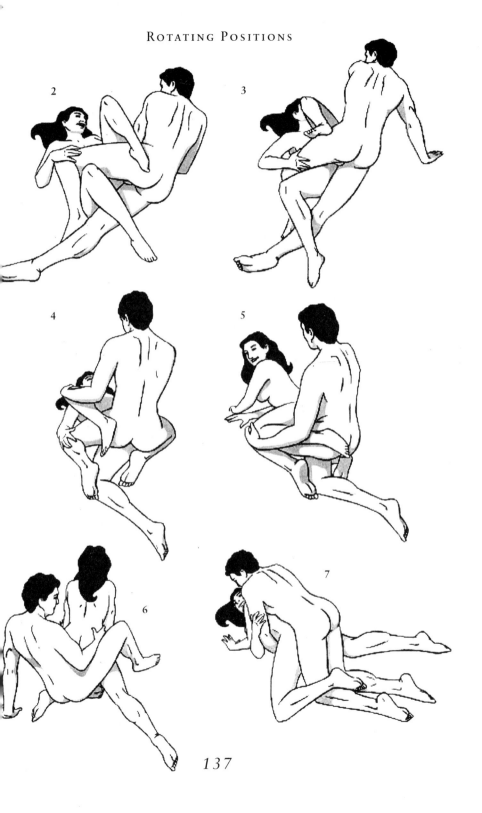

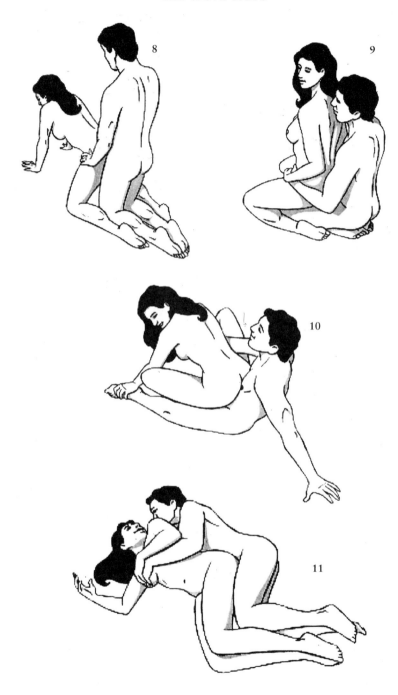

vagina, simply re-insert it and find a suitable position. Couples sometimes say to me, "This position works for me but not for him, so we are having problems." I remind them that they are a unit, that the penis and vagina make love together. So if a position does not work for one partner, it does not work for the other either. It's better to abandon that position and explore new ones. I also point out that the more often couples make love in relaxation, the softer, more supple, and less fearful the bodies become. Often they find that positions that were once difficult are suddenly easy.

Staying conscious in exploration

It is important to know that there are some positions that are simply "dangerous!" It is likely that you drop into them because of the familiarity of falling back into old excitement patterns, but they will be less than satisfying. I found when I was beginning with Tantra that whenever I was penetrated from behind, doggie style, it was so exciting I would lose my awareness. I soon realized it was happening more in my mind than in my body. Now that my presence and sexual awareness are so much stronger, I am able to enjoy that position again without getting lost in excitement or fantasy. Even so, it takes constant alertness to stay in the mysterious here and now, receiving and absorbing the flowing male energy. Many a time I chose to abandon my awareness, and roll happily and blindly down the roller coaster of excitement, having a wonderful time! But gradually I found that being present and in genital communion while in that particular position, with that particular angle of penetration, turned out to be much more ecstatic than the excitement from before.

This is perhaps the most compelling aspect of exploring sex. It is really fun to be making love all the time, slowly coming to understand what is happening, putting together a new picture. Intensity increases as different emotions start to clear out of the body, you feel more available and sensitive and because the emotions arise in the face of love, deep healing is possible. Love washes away the pains of the past, at times with tears, at times with laughter, and at times with silence.

There are certain positions that are simply comfortable, thereby encouraging long periods of lovemaking. Sometimes, it is wonderful to just plug in, close your eyes, relax back, and rest in consciousness for an hour or two *(see* fig. 13).

The scissors position earlier suggested for soft penetration (with the man lying on his side, the woman on her back, opening her legs and bringing her pelvis to his) is especially good because it *is* relatively neutral. Nobody is on top and nobody underneath; it is nicely balanced, and more important, comfortable for both. Also, most people can find it with ease, so it can be a relaxing position to start making love.

The man on the top, the classic "doing" or missionary position *(see* fig. 14), can also be used successfully for "non-doing" and deep penetration. The man simply lies forward or kneels over the woman without thrusting, keeping the penetration deep and still. The woman can raise her legs, curling her pelvis upward to facilitate the penetration. From here it is easy to roll to one side or the other as a unit, maintaining deep vaginal contact. Using pillows to make the position comfortable, the man lies between the woman's legs and the couple face each other on their sides. These positions are also good for cleansing and healing of the genitals, where deep penetration is needed.

Fig. 13   Side position: relaxed and serene with eyes closed

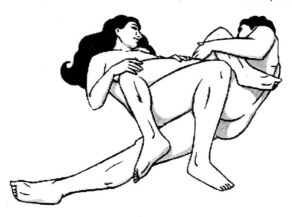

140

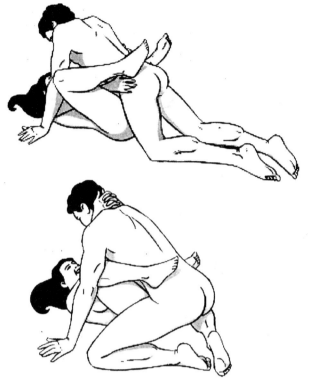

Fig. 14   Man on top position

The Yab Yum position—an ecstatic circle of energy
The sitting position, called the Yab Yum position *(see* fig. 15), is wonderful because the spine and body energy are vertical, aligned with heaven and earth, with gravitation and levitation. The chest and breasts meet easily here, as do eyes and lips and an ecstatic fulfilling circle of energy is experienced between the bodies. When you try this one out you may need a pillow under the woman's buttocks to support her pelvis, making it easier for you both to maintain this position comfortably. Do it only if it feels right. When the sexual channels are open, the sexual energy will automatically place the body in certain positions as a function of the energetic force between the bodies and not from any conscious decision.

141

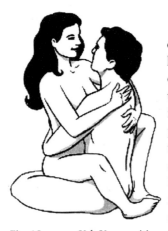

Fig. 15   Yab Yum position

There are books on sex which describe special positions said to have a magical effect, but these originated from the intelligence of two conscious bodies, and not from the mind. When these positions are turned into techniques unsupported by the awareness and sexual energy, they become empty shells of no intrinsic value. So don't worry about special positions. Instead, put your focus into the genitals while you make love, and if you feel sleepy or insensitive, change position and you will find suddenly you are more present and aware of the sexual energy. When you allow the bodies to respond to each other and dance together, the positions will take care of themselves.

KEY POINTS:

ॐ Presence and awareness are more important than positions.

ॐ The vagina and the penis within it form one unit.

ॐ Preserve this unity to increase the possibility of energetic exchange.

ॐ Change positions by rotating around the genital connection.

ॐ This naturally changes the angle of penetration to increase sensitivity.

ॐ Shifting positions bring presence, life, and dance into love.

PART
3

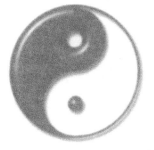

THE
JOURNEY

15

MAKE A DATE
TO MAKE LOVE

WE MAKE DINNER DATES, theater dates and business dates, but rarely lovemaking dates. For some reason making love, which is foremost in most people's thoughts, usually ends up absolutely last on the list. Most of us finish working, eating, drinking, entertaining, before we consider love. And then when exhausted, or under the effects of alcohol, or digesting a heavy meal, or all three, we decide to make love. This is hardly the time when we are at our best, so to expect such an experience to be a beautiful and sacred celebration of love is unrealistic, even unfair.

Often when we make a date for dinner or the movies, we do so with the desire to end up in bed. But there we sit, crossing and uncrossing our legs, eating course after course, plowing through conversation, wondering anxiously when it will happen, or if it will happen at all! But whenever I have had the courage to be honest with a man about what I wanted, I experienced instant relief, my energy could flow freely and this helped me to be natural.

I have always appreciated it too, when a man was direct with his intentions, when he spoke up and told me that he wanted to make love, without the game that usually preceded sex. Making a date to make love is uncommon in this society. However, many couples who have tried this approach say at first there was a resistance because it took away the spontaneity of sex, but later reported that it worked out very well. The women said that after they got over the idea that they were "making love on demand" it brought deep contentment to know that they would definitely make love with their partner. They felt more appreciated and loved, more open and available. The men reported feeling infinitely more relaxed when they knew they would be making love at a specific time, because it reduced their mental obsession with sex. They found it more easy to concentrate on other activities during the day without the repeated sexual thoughts or anxieties. Many said that knowing they had a date to make love stopped the compulsive looking at other women.

As much as people say that they want things to be spontaneous, the truth is that this seldom happens. We do the same thing in sex again and again. Men are often concerned well in advance about if and when women will allow them to make love again. Women have been known to intentionally withhold sex from their partners; we have all heard the jokes about women and their perpetual headaches that pop up at bedtime. "When will she let me inside her again?" the man asks himself, and this makes him restless and anxious. Knowing that she *will* be there, ready and willing to make love, is reassuring for the man. He knows that he will not have to win her over or persuade her, and this relaxation gives him a natural loving authority, enabling him to direct his male energy in a creative way. So it becomes important that the woman does not make up excuses when the time arrives to make love. Certainly, occasions will arise when there are genuine reasons why she cannot participate, but in general it is really worthwhile and most interesting to make love regardless of what else is going on. When the woman sticks to her commitment to make love, the man is less anxious, and this is also of benefit to him. Knowing that love will happen can serve to prolong the lovemaking too, since anxiety would create tension, which creates excitement and the likelihood of early ejaculation.

Making love without a date or preparation means that it happens by accident, which also implies with less consciousness. When I began making dates to make love, I found that knowing beforehand actually made me a more sensitive lover. I could tune into sex several hours before the event, become conscious of my breasts and my vagina slowly pulling the awareness into my body before my lover arrived. When we finally lay down together I was almost ready for penetration. The idea of cooperating together in this way, and the mental preparation that comes with it, changes the whole quality of lovemaking.

Sexual dating

It is quite possible that at first when you start "dating" in this way, you feel a little embarrassed, even shy or awkward, especially when it is time to undress and get into bed. To take this conscious step, rather than fumbling around on the sofa in a prolonged seduction, can be a challenge in itself. Nonetheless it is worth taking the plunge. Remove your clothing consciously and slowly and allow yourself to be seen. Look at each other with soft vision. Gradually approach each other, gently embrace, remembering to keep the awareness inward and downward. You may prefer to lie down facing each other, or sit opposite each other. Such honesty brings a vitality, which compels you into the experience of the present moment.

I remember a friend telling me after reading some articles I had written that he and his partner decided to make a date to make love. He was surprised to find that he felt tremendously bashful and self-conscious about it even though he had been making love with her for years. He found this so overwhelming that he decided to abandon the attempt. However, isn't it interesting that we feel embarrassed when suddenly we become conscious of what is happening? And that when sex happens by accident and in the dark we often feel more comfortable with it? As we bring the sexual act into consciousness there are likely to be some awkward moments at first, but don't be disheartened. Trust your lover, for there is no need for protection or pretense. You are here in love. As the self-consciousness dissolves we become more present and trusting. After two or three dates it will seem quite natural to approach sex in this way and you will welcome how straightforward it is.

How often should we make love?

I am often asked how often a couple should make love. I find it very healthy to make love as often as possible. When energy is generated and not dispersed, one is enriched and uplifted by the experience. One can make love again and again. It keeps your love rooted in the physical body, creating a mutual, non-mental, and energetic bond between you. This increases your awareness of each other, and times in between take on a different quality. A simple breakfast can have an underlying joy and contented silence to it while a sparkle in the eyes and a flashing smile transmit more than words can say. Intimacy is in the air and it grows.

When I began to change the way I made love, I was fortunate to be living a flexible lifestyle so I had lots of time available. I was so fascinated with the revelations of the new world I was exploring, I was grateful to find my lover as enthusiastic and available as I was, so we made love daily and more than once. This enabled it to be an organic living process and we entered into our journey freely, putting together a unique and different picture, discovering something new each time. Even when we did not really feel like making love, we still put our bodies together and it was astounding to discover that the bodies *always* loved to make love, even if the mind was not so interested. The more we made love the more we understood how and why certain results happened, and we were able to unravel the misunderstandings that held us in the old, non-satisfying patterns of our sexual past.

That was my personal experience, but ultimately we must each decide for ourselves how often making love is appropriate. Some couples value it every day because it keeps the thread of love and consciousness weaving in the body. It becomes a significant part of daily life. For others, the pressures of work and family make it impossible to come together every day. For them, once or twice a week is more realistic. Whatever your lifestyle offers is what you will do. Frequency is really not the issue; what is significant here is quality. A truly joyful sexual experience can leave you satisfied and glowing for days. Just make love as often as you can, remembering when you make love consciously, no energy will be wasted or dispersed. You will in fact be generating energy, and you will be invigorated. You might even find you begin to need less sleep.

When you make a date to make love, I suggest that you give yourself around two to three hours . . . or more. Ensure that you have no disturbances by switching on the answering machine and locking the door. Where there is a lack of privacy, anxieties can arise which will provoke sexual excitement and make it difficult to relax into the experience. If possible don't limit your lovemaking to the night; also choose times when the body is fresh and awake, preferably after some exercise, dancing, or meditation. Try dates at different times of the day to see what works best for you. Mornings are good because the day has only just started. The body is renewed after a night's sleep and the mind is relatively still, not yet filled up with daily anxieties. The afternoons are also favorite times for many lovers and if your work schedule does not allow this, try the weekends. You must make a conscious effort, even if it means sending your children to friends for the afternoon. Then instead of watching a movie, make love! Some years ago one couple, after having a two-hour talk with me, started to spend Friday mornings together. They changed their work schedules to create a few hours at home while the children were at school. It became a hallowed day and even the neighbors noticed the serene quietness surrounding the house. This weekly date helped their relationship enormously and the children in turn benefited from the happy environment created by the conscious loving of their parents.

Love in the center of your life

This does not mean that you must only make love when there

are two or three hours available. When there is little time to make love, Tantra has its own version of the sexual "quickie," which is about plugging in rather than going for it. Just slip the relaxed penis into the vagina as suggested in the section on soft penetration and lie together in consciousness for twenty minutes. Joining like this in the morning after coffee and before work can bring the fresh breeze of contentment into your day. At night, if you are sleepy but find you want to be closer to your lover, as a good-night kiss try fifteen minutes of plugging in energy exchange. You can even go to sleep like this, relaxing happily back into the night. If you are separating from your lover for a time, make a date to make love before leaving—even ten minutes works wonders. It is beautiful to say good-bye in a conscious way instead of a final few words over your shoulder at an airport gate after a sad or tearful hug.

Making a date to make love is putting love back into the center of your life as a priority. There is far less wasted time when suddenly small talk with acquaintances is less appealing, and you can't wait to get back home and dive gratefully into bed with your lover. Some couples, particularly if they have been together for many years, have found it essential to write lovemaking into their schedules, fitting it around the clamor of children, relatives, and peer-group pressures. They sit together on the weekends and make appointments with each other! Don't let the idea of two to three hours intimidate you. The important thing is to make it open-ended so that you do not have to think about the end. A full one hundred and eighty minutes means that you definitely have to arrive in the present, and be here. Have a hot bath, dance together, share massage, make love, have a cup of tea, and make love again. If it seems like nothing is happening, a short break is always a worthwhile idea. It usually works wonders, refreshing you both, and when you start again it is a whole new adventure. In this way, making a date to make love, whether it is a long time or a short one, will help to bring some focus back into your love affair. Making love whenever possible becomes a significant factor for many couples, and they soon discover that sexual rapport is the root of loving contentment. Frequency in lovemaking deepens your personal experience. It also infuses a certain stillness in the body, which is very healthy, and even life's activities have a more centered quality. This frequency also reduces the tremendous pressure of expectations we have surrounding the sexual act, which interfere with our capacity to be present. We find it much easier to "be" when we make love often. We are relaxed and easy and whatever happens is what happens. With this unexpecting attitude, exploration and discovery are possible.

Create an atmosphere of intimacy

It may be that you need time to talk, to share the events of the day or any unclear feelings which you are experiencing. Clear and share these before you begin to make love, because unspoken anxieties and concerns will distract you from the present moment with your lover. Unexpressed feelings in particular act as a subtle screen between you and your lover, preventing deeper energetic intimacy. The mind fights hard to rationalize itself out of sharing feelings, but sexual energy responds to honesty. Many couples have found that psychological openness leads to increased physical ecstasy. Tantra reminds us to make love only when in a loving and sharing mood, suggesting that if you are feeling in the least argumentative, don't be in a hurry to use sex to bring you together. It is better to relax together and massage each other, getting clear and cool and creating the intimacy again as you come down to earth. Then make love much, much later.

When you make a date to make love it gives you a chance to experiment with the Love Keys, and you now have a variety of suggestions to try out. Whatever you remember is what is best for you to use as you start experimenting. And whatever works for you is a key for you. It may not be a suggestion included here but if it helps you to be more present, it is your key. You can have many keys which you use simultaneously—breathing, eye contact, consciousness of the positive pole, while relaxing the feet. There are an infinite number of keys to help shift the consciousness inward, and as you become more sensitive the keys become more subtle.

KEY POINTS:

ह≈ Agreeing on a time to make love puts love back in your life.

ह≈ It increases relaxation, consciousness, and commitment.

ह≈ Each meeting is an opportunity to experiment with the Love Keys.

ह≈ The more we make love, the more we wish to make love.

ह≈ The well-used words "making love" regain their original meaning as we feel the influence of love in our lives.

16

FOREPLAY AFRESH

WARMING UP TO LOVEMAKING is essential so that our energies can awaken and slowly attune to each other. It gives time for a natural attraction to arise, and this makes all the difference. It is good for both men and women, but especially women. Since women represent the negative polarity, they need and appreciate the time prior to penetration to be fully available for love. And it must be a loving and gentle play, not a serious business with goals in mind as if following a mechanical manual.

In a fresh approach to making love, the most significant thing about foreplay is that it should not produce too much excitement. Don't make your partner too excited, even though it may be tempting at times. This makes it difficult to move into a relaxing sexual experience. When desire or lust is provoked through sexual stimulation, the energy moves toward release. As a result, staying conscious in and aware of the present moment will be difficult. In the Tantric approach to foreplay, it is the attitude of the mind that is most important. How you do it, not what you do, is the point. If you wish to make your partner hot and horny this requires a particular attitude and approach, a certain intention. How and where you touch will make all the difference. However, a man who really takes the time to gently awaken the body of a woman through a slow, sensual approach will feel the inviting environment once penetration occurs.

Rediscovering erogenous zones

Nature gave us erogenous zones that function naturally to produce sexual interest and excitation. Excitation can be felt as the buzzing of life energy itself and this is not to be confused with excitement. These erogenous zones assist us in accessing our life energy, and they function as bridges to the present moment. However, through our lack of understanding in sex we overuse or abuse our erogenous zones, and they gradually become desensitized. This may show up as a lack of sensitivity where we withdraw physically and close down to the other and thus ourselves, or it may reflect as hypersensitivity, where we become unbearably sensitive, almost repelled by touch. The body can also feel leaden, numb, and dead.

For example, a woman's nipples can become either dull and unresponsive or extremely sensitive to touch, almost painful. The tendency to either reaction is to immediately push the other person away. The same thing can happen to the clitoris, especially if used habitually to achieve orgasm. An insensitive touch can also have a repelling effect and will cause a woman to withdraw sexually at the very moment that her partner is trying to reach her.

In Tantra we learn that the breasts and nipples are a woman's positive pole, the gateway to her sexual expression, and she can be brought to the depths and heights of orgasm through her breasts. The breasts are the route to her feminine sexual energy. So it becomes meaningful for a woman to have sensitivity in her breasts, and to be able to welcome and receive attention there. She must not react to the touch but respond and open up to it, so a man must take care how he touches her.

A useful guideline is to see if the approach contracts or expands your body energy, noticing whether it leads to more excitement and tension, or more inner sensitivity and expansion. It is beautiful and natural for a woman to touch the penis, but usually when she does so she wants it to be erect immediately so penetration and orgasm can happen. The classic way to get an erection going is to use friction by moving the hand backward and forward. With this kind of stimulation, the man will feel excited, restless, and desirous of moving once he is inside the woman, making it more difficult for him to penetrate slowly and consciously. With masturbation-like movements, the penis feels an unspoken pressure and demand for an erection, sometimes making it more difficult for him to achieve. This type of erection, which relies on stimulation, can be temperamental, fragile, and easy to lose, so once the man is inside the woman he will then have to continuously maintain and build up the level of sexual excitement in order to remain erect. In this way sex can become frenzied and overexciting, leading to quick ejaculation.

When the penis is fondled and caressed unhurriedly without the intention to get an erection, where the touch is loving and not demanding, this can be a beautiful experience, a wonderful sharing of energy. When the woman simply touches the penis with loving presence, when she massages, squeezes, pulls the foreskin folds back, the penis will absorb the love, feel the interest, and respond accordingly. The erection will be a side-effect of the love, with a different quality than that experienced when erection arises from a mental or physical pressure. The intention here is to love and adore the penis for its wonderful qualities, a healing, loving power tool. The penis itself recognizes the difference in the woman's attitude and feels empowered.

Relax to expand energy and extend your lovemaking

Playing with excitement is a natural phenomenon, a delightful energy, but use the excitation just enough to warm you up and light the fire and then relax into the joy of it. Tantric sex and conventional sex are similar in the beginning, when some life and a flame of attraction is needed. But here the similarity ends because Tantra stays with the beginning. It can be prolonged for hours if you wish. In conventional sex, where excitement is built up, the fire that we started will soon become dying coals. The wind rushes through and burns the fire so rapidly that for many people sex lasts only a few minutes. Tantra discourages action that fans the fire, causing it to burn too quickly. Instead we stay within the flames of the initial attraction, fanning them with awareness and presence. The fire will gradually engulf the whole body, keeping it glowing and radiant for hours. You feel as if you are floating beneath excitement, keeping yourself alert to the needs of each moment. If a little excitement is needed to maintain the erection, stimulate yourself in some way, perhaps by moving, but only for a few moments. Then relax again, staying cool and extending the lovemaking so that the energy flows fully, bringing deep satisfaction. When couples are able to achieve this kind of sexual union, they find themselves more loving with each other and cooperation is a natural outcome in their daily lives.

Become aware of your partner's response as you touch and caress. Avoid going places that make your lover too excited, or try touching the same place but in a different way. Because the vagina and clitoris have long since and mistakenly been the center of stimulating attention during foreplay, it is better to do something soft and acknowledging rather than vigorous. The clitoris for example, when touched with rapid movements, creates a great deal of excitement. Try gently resting your fingers on it, doing nothing, just touching. If you move your finger do it slowly. Or try placing the whole hand over the pubic bone, cupping it very lightly, and hold it there for several minutes without doing anything active. Send energy and love through your hand. Softly touching, pulling, and playing with the pubic hair can be a nice turn-on, or a gentle tapping on the pubic bone feels great. In general, soft, considerate touch expands the body energy and makes you more sensitive—it is an instant turn-on, while pressured or rough, demanding touch causes the body to shrink and contract and harden in defense, making it less receptive.

Oral sex in foreplay

By now you may be asking yourself about the wonders of oral sex in foreplay. Many people have come to rely on it as an integral part of the sexual act, but because the interaction of penis in vagina alone does not satisfy deeply its ecstatic potential is unknown. However, oral stimulation of the penis and clitoris produces a great deal of excitement and reduces the consciousness of the genitals. Both men and women have found that oral sex desensitizes the penis and vagina, and ruins the profound effects of simple conscious penetration. And now with our information about polarity, positive and negative, we can see that there is virtually nô bio-electric alignment between mouths and genitals. While oral sex may be exciting, the deeper energies are not awakened, and once the ecstatic magnetic function of the penis and vagina are tasted, oral sex can eventually cease to be of interest, or enjoyed occasionally just for fun.

For women, the question of lubrication arises in the context of foreplay. Usually lubrication is achieved through stimulation of some kind but because we are avoiding this, it is better to use a lubricant or saliva. Apply a little at the entrance of the vagina, then some on the penis itself. Spreading it on in a slow and sensual way from the head down to the root can be fun, making it part of foreplay, so don't be embarrassed to suggest it. Men are more than willing to use it, as it helps them to slide effortlessly into the woman, and they thoroughly enjoy the application of it! Remember to spread it on in a way that brings life, not hunger, to the penis. The idea is to lubricate, not agitate.

A woman is likely to find after making love in a relaxed way her vagina will lubricate itself more easily. As the vagina and surrounding tissues relax and become more sensitive and responsive, less stimulation is required. A relaxed vagina is smooth and moist in general, so only a small amount of lubricant is needed here and on the head of the penis to facilitate penetration.

Touching breasts and chest

Most women long for their breasts to be touched and loved because it unites their upper and lower parts bringing a deep sexual fulfillment. Caressing the breasts overflows warmth and aliveness into the vagina. But in contrast, when the breasts are

157

strongly squeezed or sucked and over stimulated, this can have the effect of rapidly agitating or exciting a woman, urging her to achieve orgasm. This can have the tendency to flip her over the edge, from feeling to frenzy in a few seconds flat! The response of the nipples in this case is not a true one, but rather a conditioned reaction that gives birth to tension, lust, and sexual expectation. The authentic response of the breasts and nipples has the effect of expanding the body energy, softening of the heart, and showering an overflow of warm life into the vagina. It is nothing to do with getting something; it helps you to be increasingly here, more passionate, more present.

Tell your lover how to touch your breasts and nipples and this will help you both enormously. A woman should encourage her partner to touch her breasts in a way that she is able to receive and absorb his touch. The greater the depth of feeling in her breasts, the more open her heart, and the deeper the sexual energy responds. A woman ought not rely entirely on her partner to awaken her positive pole, and it is highly recommended that she begins to cultivate awareness in the breasts from within herself. During lovemaking and at other times, she is encouraged to "hold" her breasts in the forefront of her awareness (both nipples simultaneously), filling them with energy, melting into them so as to activate her own body electricity. And while making love, a woman can touch her own breasts to nourish this awareness.

Many men are sensitive in their nipples too, and enjoy being touched here. When you do so, include the entire chest and heart area in your caress, stroking the chest, feeling its furry or silky muscular textures. Include touching an important pressure point in the center of the chest, sometimes called the Love Spot, lying on the breast bone directly in line with the nipples. Massaging this point firmly in a circular motion stimulates the thymus gland and the immune system while it warms and opens the heart. When the chest area of a man is activated through loving touch or his own awareness, it helps him to be more considerate and conscious as he makes love, his heart too, feels acknowledged. When chest and breasts meet, a man can imagine himself receiving energy of woman through his heart, and can allow his heart to be penetrated with love.

Breathing and kissing

If you breathe consciously slowly and deeply as you approach your lover during foreplay it makes for tremendous sensuality. Breathing in and out of your mouth can bring you in tune with your body and in harmony with your partner. As you touch or are being touched, breathe deeply into the hands, feel the breath wrapping and penetrating the cells with consciousness. Be adventurous with your breathing, it activates the life energy and encourages you to be fully present in your body.

Kissing is a truly wonderful and sensual art, and it can become a language in itself, an important aspect of foreplay and lovemaking. It evokes the sexual response at a deep level. Kissing, being joined at the mouth, is the ultimate intimacy of face-to-face and eye-to-eye. It is an extremely intimate gesture and often a person will think once about making love with someone, but think twice about kissing them. It is as if we consider kissing to be more sacred than sex. If we are in love, as we make love, then there is usually the overwhelming wish to kiss each other. It is a profound sharing of energy, a drinking through the sensuality of the mouth, and through this the bodies connect in intimate circular fullness.

However, in kissing as in lovemaking, once again we do too much. Relaxation is the biggest aid to kissing. Relax the mouth and jaw and especially relax the lips, allowing them to be soft and receptive. Usually in kissing we purse the lips into a tight rosebud and then we kiss the other person on their tightened lips very quickly. This is not really a genuine kiss, one where there is a sharing of energy through the mouth because the lips are too tense. Lips need to be relaxed and pliable, yielding and responsive. In kissing, bring the lips together very very slowly; let them join softly, be elastic, melt into each other. Maintain this juicy contact allowing them to answer each other in a succulent dance.

Today much emphasis is given to tongue kissing, the famous

French kiss. However, in Tantra this is maintained for special occasions when the sex energy is flowing deeply. At the onset of kissing, a tongue thrust in the mouth of a woman can easily have an off-putting effect. It is too much too soon, she needs a slower approach. Kissing with the tongue can also trigger excitement very quickly, especially in the case of a man. So during foreplay and lovemaking this is something to watch for if you wish to keep the sexual temperature cool. The thrusting tongue is often used by men as a substitute for the penis, especially when it is not possible to penetrate the woman, and also where he feels his penis to be inadequate.

At first, when leaving the tongue out of kissing, it can seem a little strange or incomplete, but soon you are able to feel the thrill and sensuality of the succulent lips themselves. Penetrate your lips with your presence and awareness, and you will be amazed at the effects in your own body and in your partner's response. In approaching love, enjoy a sense of humor, be childlike and innocent, unknowing and fresh. Lie together, cuddle and kiss and even rub noses!

Separating in consciousness

It is good to realize that separating slowly and respectfully is as important and significant as coming together slowly and respectfully. Foreplay and afterplay are one and the same thing. Conscious lovemaking creates a very powerful energy field around a couple, and if suddenly disrupted it can be extremely disturbing, producing quite the opposite effect. The intimate exchange creates a deep bonding, nurturing and healing. It can be a physical and psychological shock when, for example, the man suddenly and unexpectedly withdraws his penis from the vagina leaving the woman with the feeling of being unplugged or suddenly abandoned by her lover, and the benefits experienced from the lovemaking can easily be destroyed. The energy fields are one, so avoid sudden separation. Tell your partner when you wish to separate your bodies, and do it slowly and consciously.

After making love it is really worthwhile to lie down side by side in consciousness, and relax together in silence after sexual union. Keep your attention inward before scattering the energy with talking or laughing, focusing on the streaming sensations in the body. This strongly reinforces your sensitivity and consciousness and has transforming effects.

KEY POINTS

꿈A woman's body warms up slowly and appreciates loving foreplay.

꿈Keep the sexual temperature cool; it's not what we do, but how we do it.

꿈A slow, conscious approach expands the body energies.

꿈Include the positive poles, especially the breasts.

꿈Breathing, kissing, and touching awaken the senses.

17

PLEASING AND
PERFORMANCE

W E ALL WONDER IF WE ARE GOOD LOVERS.
"Do I please my partner?" we ask ourselves. "And
am I good enough or am I too much?" We want to be
valued and enjoyed which puts pressure on us in bed. We want
to do it right, make it work. But because the emphasis has been
placed on the outcome, the end result, it has also led to
performing and pleasing. When we have an idea of what should
happen and we do our best to engineer that event, we are not in
contact with our core, the source of the sex energy. The energy,
instead of heating up and expanding inside each of us, gets
directed or leaked outward in pleasing and performance.

Due to our physical differences, the brunt of performance
pressure falls on the man. Since he has to maintain a full
erection every time for intercourse to take place, he has an
enormous burden to carry. When men share their feelings about
desperate nights where every attempt for erection failed, you
can feel their tremendous pain. It is not surprising that men
suffer anxiety, because without this miraculous phenomenon
we are not able to penetrate and make love, which further
creates the concept of performance.

This concept dictates that the man has to perform well, do a
good show, give her a good ride, an attitude that suggests that

in order to be a good lover, a man must be a good machine. This results in the man directing himself to "doing," making something happen, and this has made him mechanical. He believes he must get as hard as possible as soon as possible, and so he directs his energy outward in his desire for the outward projection of his penis. This takes him away from his bodily consciousness, from his ability to relax and trust in his body. The belief is that a man *has* to act in some way for love to happen. But in order to embrace a new style of lovemaking, we must make a fundamental shift by pulling the attention back to ourselves. The emphasis on the penis being hard for love is one of the most basic misunderstandings between lovers. The truth is, when the penis finds itself in loving, relaxed sexual surroundings, he will grow erect easily or, at least, hard enough for penetration. And remember the delightful possibility of soft penetration where no erection is needed. A man in one of my groups once said, "When my penis is soft, I don't even consider it to be a penis." This is not so. Hard or soft, the penis is always infused with energy.

Forget the performance, be in the awareness

For a man sex has become so much an aspect of the mind, and he has been so busy monitoring his performance or been in fantasy to stimulate performance, he has rarely had the chance to really feel down into his penis. He's been around it and using it, but not truly in it. Now with this new orientation, where performance is no longer required, he can re-direct his energy into feeling the marvel that he has between his legs. He can start to feel that he is his penis inside the vagina, in fact and not fantasy. When he merges his consciousness with his penis, it becomes incredibly sensitive and perceptive, and this has nothing to do with performance and nothing to do with size. When the genitals are viewed as a single unit and experienced as generative organs, sensitivity is an asset, not size. Men have reported that many of the usual feelings of competition between men, the parading of physical prowess, fell away once they embraced a new way of making love.

The woman, because she does not need an erection, is not challenged to perform in the same way as a man. She knows she must get wet, but dryness is easily overcome. Lubricant or saliva will do, so the performance pressure on woman is far less. In knowing that without an erection she cannot have her man, however, she will begin to perform to please him. She is notorious for faking her orgasms. She may pretend too, through sounds and movements, that she is enjoying the way her man is touching her or thrusting inside her even when she is not, simply because she hopes she is turning him on, and hoping he will stay harder for a longer time. Most women have done this, and some have even suffered physical pain during intercourse, but they ignore it. Instead they stay focused on pleasing the man to support his performance instead of being aware of what is happening in their own body. Is my vagina relaxed? What if I stopped moving backward and forward? How about letting him in deeper? Changing the angle of my pelvis? A woman will notice as she brings consciousness to herself during sex, that many of her movements are oriented toward the man and pleasing his penis, rather than toward herself, and her receptivity in her vagina. Tantra informs us that when a woman's vagina is relaxed, the penis will grow erect naturally. Where the environment is yielding and porous, there is more likelihood of attraction and response.

When a woman's energy is swinging away from herself in pleasing, and a man's energy is projected outward in performance, there can be no genuine exchange of sexual energy between opposite poles. Rather, both are off center and away from home and more likely to have an explosive quick bang than the long, slow, sensual burn envisaged by Tantra.

We all know that if a fire has too much air and wood, it burns too quickly. We also know if it has no air or wood, it won't burn at all. A fire needs exactly the right amount of wood and air to keep it glowing into the early hours. If we compare this to lovemaking, we can realize how much love and understanding is needed to keep a continual awareness on the wood and flow of air.

Excitement is what we have been taught to use to get us where we want to go. This "heat" stokes us up prior to penetration. Once the penis is inside, we need even more heat to maintain the erection. In creating a quick fire, stoking it up as much as possible, we make it burn all the more fiercely. But more important, when we create the heat in another person's body before creating it in ourselves, we are making a false fire.

Experience your body from within

When you slowly withdraw projection, forgetting about the other person and coming back to yourself, the relationship to your own body will become extremely significant. You can concentrate on relaxing, breathing, and experiencing your body from within. When you stop thinking about the other person, over whom you have no real influence anyway, and bring your attention back home, you are stoking your own fire.

You must look after yourself first before tending to the fire that belongs to someone else. Then you will be in for a big surprise! When your fire is alight, reach out to your lover. Keep lighting your fire as you come closer, and if they have lit theirs, there is the potential for glowing golden embers. Keep asking yourself, "Am I doing this for me, or some idea I have about me?" and this will provide invaluable answers. The moment you find yourself projecting outward, pleasing or performing, drop back into your own center, and usually you will both experience a wave of sexual energy coursing through your bodies.

The time for penetration is always a delicate moment and the pressures of pleasing and performing can easily manifest here. Often when the bodies and energies are prepared for penetration, the minds are preoccupied with concerns *about* penetration. Is it too soon? Is it going to happen? Will it work? Will she let me in? Frequently a man will penetrate his partner before she is physically or psychologically prepared which can lead to the woman feeling forced and therefore resistant to making love. To reduce these pressures and to increase consciousness it is important that a woman is willing to be penetrated. I suggest to couples that as soon as the woman is ready she invites her partner to enter her. If the man is erect, well and good, if he is not, more time is needed and the woman can wait. Or you may agree to try soft penetration. The man with his active positive pole of love is naturally more likely to be ready while the woman is sexually more passive and usually needs more time than her man. When the woman invites penetration she enters as a willing and responsive partner. It must be added, however, that the woman must not withhold penetration from her man as part of a push-and-pull power game. This will bring in the element of the mind and its desire to control the other, and this attitude has no place in the Tantric approach to love. Partners attempting to create a new basis for their love should enter into lovemaking with sincerity and honesty.

Women and men find the suggestion that a woman proposes penetration very helpful. Men like it because it puts the responsibility with the woman, he can relax and not worry about the perfect moment to approach her. Women appreciate it too. She can now relax without the pressure to force herself into readiness through excitement. It is clear that entry is up to her and there is no possibility of violating boundaries. When a woman welcomes him into her vagina, a man will feel the difference and it is worth the wait.

You will find that soon the penis and vagina become attuned to this new approach as increased sensitivity arises and the pressures to please and perform die down. Lie together for a few minutes, allow the eyes to meet, have a few breaths, relax, and you are both ready. It is as if the organs understand that love is being handed over to them now. Their intrinsic response to each other is activated as they sense the responsibility of love now lies with them. In normal circumstances mental pressure inhibits this natural response. Gradually, very subtle phenomena become more than enough to awaken sexual energy without needing to please or perform for the other.

Pleasing and appearances

We find ourselves today in a tragically body-beautiful society, and women in particular find an obsessive pressure placed on them to conform to its stringent demands. Again this leads us to an objective and external view of ourselves, and we lose connection to our inner world, our subjectivity, the source of our beauty. True radiant beauty has little to do with physical features. It is a quality that shimmers from within. When a woman is fulfilled in love she is extremely beautiful, even luminous, with love. It shines through the physical form. The inspiring curves of feminine grace are to be found in every woman's body. Awareness and a loving attitude to one's own body plant the roots of real beauty, elegance, and dignity. Yet most of us judge or compare rather than love our bodies. Forget about the norm, and start to love your body from within while appreciating the shapes and forms of others. Acceptance and relaxation have a profound effect on the body energy, which creates unique feminine beauty.

KEY POINTS:

ॐ Forget about being a perfect lover—without a goal there is nothing to prove.

ॐ Redirect that same energy into feeling your own body from within.

ॐ When a man and a woman are relaxed and receptive, loving is easy.

ॐ The radiance of love is the true source of beauty in a woman.

18

ORGASM AND EJACULATION

ORGASM IS AN IMPORTANT TOPIC in the Tantric context, a discussion that becomes heated easily. In conventional sex, there is little question about it; ejaculation and orgasm are the primary reasons for making love. They are relaxing and disperse tensions, they help us to sleep well and they are both most enjoyable sensations. When you take them away it seems that there is no reward, that the fun is being removed. For many men and for some women, sex without ejaculation is inconceivable.

But after a man ejaculates, sex is over. The opportunity for closeness and sharing energy has passed, simply evaporated. This is exactly where Tantra says, "'Why end it here?" Why come and throw out your semen habitually? It is pure energy, it is imbued with the potency of life force, so keep it inside yourself. The body will ejaculate if it really has to ejaculate; you don't need to help it along.

Many men report feeling depleted after ejaculation. The jokes in our society about men turning over and snoring after they come are actually sad but true. And yet we still go for the end of the sex act. There is little doubt that through our conditioning, our lovemaking has the tendency to be outcome-oriented. The urgency of restless excitement motivates us, filling us with the desire to be rid of an inner tension. During sex if we don't achieve an orgasm or have an ejaculation we feel as if nothing happened. It was not a satisfying or real sexual experience. You may find yourself discontent, irritable, or argumentative, feeling like you were cheated, that you were at the mercy of your lover's whims and wishes, especially if your partner came and you did not.

We become addicted to orgasm and ejaculation because through them we release our internal pressures. It feels good but have you ever asked yourself how you really feel about the need for an orgasm, aside from the pure and simple enjoyment? Do you really *have to come*? Do you feel that you have made love even if you do not come? Being identified or attached to the experience of coming makes it difficult to move in the Tantric way because you have somewhere to go with a fixed idea in mind. According to the principles of Tantra there is nothing to do with nowhere to go. It is within this orientation that the Tantric experience most easily arises.

A peak experience—a circle of desire and release

Orgasm and ejaculation are peak experiences. They come from a deliberate build up of sexual energy toward a release, something that happens more or less the same way every time. It discourages creativity in lovemaking because as the intense desire or urge for orgasm arises, we are propelled forcefully forward by the mere thought of it. And intentionally we step up the ladder of excitement, where every cell in the body, every thought in the mind, is geared toward more and more. The focus is solely on the genital sensations, and friction is used to build and intensify this. This is hard and determined work toward a short-lived heaven as sexual tension consumes the body, spills over and discharges in release. It is precisely this unconscious thrust toward orgasm that keeps the sexual experience narrow and hollow, creating an insurmountable obstacle to more joy and ecstasy. This strong urge for orgasm seems to us to be so natural but only because we are unaware of the severity of our sexual conditioning.

The conditioning (mind) that has created the desire for climax overrides the intelligence (body) of our true sexual nature, which is based on deep-seated polarity. Notice the tension and contraction in your body when it goes for the orgasm. Notice the tightening of your buttocks, the contracting of your pelvic floor and belly. And often, after coming, you feel further apart from your lover, as though the two of you have been separated suddenly. The inviting sparks that flew through the air have disappeared and a shadow hangs over you. "What was that all about?" we might ask ourselves. The truth is that the idea of coming can have the effect of going, creating frustration and unhappiness for many lovers. Again and again we return feeling empty and incomplete, and so more desire is created. We find ourselves in a vicious, restless circle of desire and release, seldom the privilege of true sexual union.

A woman is not usually able to achieve a decent climax in a short period of time. She is slower than a man, and the reason is that her sexuality is total, diffused all over her body, it includes her breasts. So unless she can go into a sexual dance while making love she will not be able to have an orgasm naturally. It needs time and relaxation. Countless women live sadly under the lifetime illusion that they are non-orgasmic. The phantom of orgasm hangs over women's heads. Many a woman has faked her orgasms and never really had one, let alone a multiple one. Women's magazines are flooded with articles about the difficulties of orgasm. The root of the problem is that women get much too tense while making love, and this is made worse by the effort of trying to come and focusing on the clitoris. The ecstatic waves of orgasm that radiate through the body, the heightened vaginal sensitivity that arises when we melt into the breasts, where we make no effort and almost bottom-out, is not something to be forced or hunted after. It requires presence. An orgasm achieved through building up the excitement through friction and stimulating the clitoris gives rise to a release of sexual tension and not the experience of sexual ecstasy possible through vaginal contact with the penis. Some of us are better at getting tense than others, some of us are better at relaxing while getting tense than others, but what we know as an orgasm is not actually the real thing!

As women get older their wish to force or push for a sexual release diminishes because it is seldom worth the effort, and this is mistakenly interpreted as a loss of interest in sex. When women hear that they do not have to orgasm, indeed they should even forget about orgasm, they are overwhelmingly relieved. It means their sex life can continue because they can finally relax. Many will say they knew intuitively that orgasm could not be the whole picture. Women can benefit too, from ignoring the clitoris and letting it come into play as and when it is stimulated by the natural contact of the bodies. When we forget about orgasm as a goal we can better access our essential orgasmic nature.

In men, the opposite problem is more prevalent since they often ejaculate too soon, whether it be within fifteen, twenty, or twenty-five minutes. But premature ejaculation at five seconds or thirty minutes after penetration is still premature. It is simply not enough time to tap and activate the exquisite sexual energies of woman or for man to derive real sexual satisfaction. The truth is that the bodies are designed to make love for many hours without aim or goal, and orgasm and ejaculation can happen or not. It is your choice and not a habit.

Relax and stay in the now

In Tantra we reduce the excitement and forget about any outcome, trusting that there is more to sex than momentary pleasure. There certainly is. It may not yet be your realm of experience, but when we relax into sexual energy, we give ourselves the choice of retaining the energy inside the body. In an attempt to break the mechanical aspect of orgasm and ejaculation, ask yourself these questions: "Where am I now? Am I focused on this moment or on the next? Am I able to feel this stroke, this penetration, or am I thinking about the next, and the next and the next?" The answer will arrive in a flash!

Ask these questions often as you make love, and notice how your attention is either on your lover's pleasure or achieving your orgasm. Notice that being slightly ahead of yourself is not the same as being present now, and learning the disparity between the two makes all the difference. Pull the focus inward and down into your center, and return to consciousness. Now radiate this awareness out from deep within, pushing yourself into the here and now through your body to meet your lover.

The question often arises that since a woman does not lose life-giving semen, why on earth shouldn't she come? If she is completely relaxed it is fine. Otherwise it is essential to understand the interconnection of the partners making love. If a woman is focused on building up an orgasm through excitement, it is quite difficult for a man to be disinterested in ejaculation. This is a basic conflict of interests within the genitals. The intensity of the woman's excitement (tension) will overwhelm the relaxation of the man and suddenly he is excited too, ready to ejaculate. When the vaginal environment gets tense, so does the penis. Even if a man is able to relax through his partner's climax, she will quite possibly find herself less interested and not so enthusiastic as she was a few moments ago. Suddenly there has been a dissipation, a leaking of energy, and the fire has fizzled out. More important, when a woman is focused on orgasm she is absent and not truly present and receptive.

The secret of Tantra is, as always, relaxation. Think about what might happen if you didn't go for a peak but instead relaxed into the valley and became a wave in the ocean. When you allow the body to relax, you reach to the source of your sex energy where you begin to move from your polarities, and much more happens. There is nothing wrong with sexual release, it is biological, but when we allow it to carry us along, overwhelm us, we forget about the journey of love that comes with it. Focusing on the peak causes us to forget about extending the ride. It's the difference between a sports car roaring through the forest, missing everything but its own momentum, and a slow, easy, contented walk through nature, smelling, tasting, and feeling everything along the way. When we pay attention to the small steps that make up the whole, we become immersed in the path, and leave the end to itself. Then it is different every time.

Choose a new way to make love

Tantra offers us the opportunity to experiment with life energy. It is not about making rules and telling you not to do things. It is saying, "You've done it the other way so many times. How about trying something different for a few months? If you don't like it, nothing is lost. In the meantime, let's play a little and see what happens. Maybe the ancient lovers who embodied and conveyed Tantra knew something you didn't."

Tantra gives you the possibility to choose a new way to make love, based on the understanding that habitual ejaculation requires a man to operate outside of his male polarity. This undermines his masculinity as he continually forces his sex energy to a peak, creating an overly positive environment within, which results in an imbalance. This leaves him more often than not debilitated and unloving. Some men accept this, thinking that the tiredness and sense of separation following sex is the name of the game, while others resent it, which gives them the impetus to explore their hidden potential. If a man is able to bring his intelligence to bear on his sexual expression, he opens up a nourishing world within himself and his partner that goes way beyond fulfilling ambitions and filling time. Men have told me that when the frequency of ejaculation is reduced they have more zest for life and a corresponding increase in sexual interest. It is not the other way around. His attraction does not fizzle out as usual, but instead it continues and grows while he feels grounded and charged with life, confidence, and a new kind of loving manliness.

Man's ejaculation is not really an orgasm, although for men the words orgasm and ejaculation are used interchangeably to describe the experience. The semen is just the physical part, but the psychic and spiritual part of orgasm is missed completely. Here is where the highest potential of sex lies. Orgasm is a state where body is no longer felt as matter; it vibrates like energy, like electricity, filled with light. You are without physical boundaries, a dancing, throbbing energy, consumed with the divine. The body becomes vaporous, vibrating in harmony with the beloved, hearts beating together, and then orgasm happens— two become one—a circle pulsating together. This is the ancient symbol of yin and yang, yin moving into yang and yang moving into yin. It is exactly this spiritual state that we are unknowingly seeking in our conventional thirst for orgasm, because in the few seconds of orgasm that we do have, we can yield to a higher force.

An inner ecstatic phenomenon

Tantra offers an orgasm that is a state and not an event. It is interested in *being* orgasmic, rather than *having* an orgasm. One is timeless and the other the fewest of seconds. This ecstatic state is an inner phenomenon from which great joy and fulfillment arises. It is the experience of a valley orgasm, a falling into the ecstatic depths of relaxation. And perhaps out of this a peak can arise from the depths, forging and swirling its way upward orgasmically to its zenith. In this valley of relaxation a man can experience orgasm without ejaculation. The orgasmic energy moves through the body in waves, but there is no physical part to it—the semen remains in the body. And women are known to release copious liquid, a divine nectar called "amrita", in moments of ecstasy.

One cannot actively seek a valley orgasm, that is its beauty. It is not a doing, it is a by-product arising out of an intensity of being, profound relaxation. It happens to you, you do not make it happen. We can actively take steps to relax in sex through the Love Keys and give birth to the possibility of such an emerging experience. And the simplest way to approach it is to resist our habit of always going for orgasm or ejaculation. Relax, remain present, and see what happens instead. It does not mean that you never come. It means you extend the lovemaking and save the ejaculation for much later on, or you come less often, and perhaps gradually with less frequency. A variety of enriching and fulfilling experiences begin to engage you and fill out the lovemaking, and correspondingly the interest or dependence on the peak recedes. It depends on you, remembering when we don't release the sex energy we are literally empowering ourselves.

When you are able to feel the *exact* moment a desire for orgasm or ejaculation arises, it is a significant and inspiring step. If you can observe the very moment when the excitement overwhelms and suddenly floods you, almost as a substance to be felt in the body, enticing you onward, *then* you can really begin to play with your sexual energy. Recognizing this precise point gives you choice in making love. The obvious choice would be to go with the desire and build it up. If you do this, do it as consciously as possible right to the end.

The less obvious choice is to relax and this is not easy. It's a confrontation with biology and conditioning, but it gives a newfound freedom. The *very instant* you feel desire, relax! And don't delay a second. In supporting the urge for even thirty seconds the desire is motivated toward release, and regaining presence becomes difficult because lust keeps kicking in. Instead, to experience the full benefit of this powerful Tantric guideline, the very instant you feel desire, face it with your full consciousness in your totality, and abandon it then and there. Drop into your body by releasing all tension—jaw, shoulders, belly, feet, wherever, let go! Relaxation flows all over the body. For men, focusing the awareness either on the third eye or the solar plexus helps in re-directing the energy. With this internal relaxation and the pressure *off* the sex energy, it inverts and moments later will rise up within, a moving force flooding you with energy, the deeper the relaxation the higher the thrust. Excitement is transformed into a thrilling energy. Riding and relaxing with this force is the art of Tantra. It becomes an inspiration, a meditation, a reason to live and love. So if you can begin to enter with consciousness, to catch the moment when the body starts to run its program and then relax intensely, the sexual energy starts to get veered off the conditioned course. It begins to valley out and expand, and you are in for a glorious surprise. Keep relaxing and you will find relaxation to be the most exciting thing around!

When you do ejaculate, experimenting with the Love Keys is worthwhile. The quality of the experience is influenced through the consciousness. Tell your partner, "I am going to come now." This acknowledgment brings immediate attention to the process. Look into her eyes. Share the energy through the eyes. Don't keep it to yourself. Relax the buttocks, the muscles at the base of the penis, slow down the movement, even try being still. Doing this will expand the experience.

Afterward, don't separate but remain lying together, embracing, penis in vagina. Keep the awareness on the genitals and allow them to exchange energy while resting. Often, when a man starts to come, the woman will intensify her efforts to achieve orgasm at the same time, but this rarely works out, it is always a few strokes short. So it is better for the woman to relax and be loving, to focus on receiving the male energy into her. If her vagina is soft and receptive, this changes the experience for the man too. In a relaxed, undemanding environment his penis will feel more alive with expanded sensations.

Discover the joy of going nowhere

After a time, making love without following our urges gets easier. You will notice that the more "here" you can be, the more enchanting the lovemaking will be. After more time, it begins to seem more natural to be "here," and the idea of coming seems like a great effort. At a certain point it feels like you step under your conditioning, beneath the superficial elements of sex, to reach a more relaxed yet vibrant state. It becomes easier to leave it up to the bodies to make love without the mind imposing a specific direction. And you do not lose your capacity to get excited and have a conventional orgasm and ejaculation. You can turn it on at any time if you so wish. The resulting peak experience of excitement is *also* an expression of the body. There are other options and choices but these only become clear to us when we start to relax into our sexual energy and give it an opportunity to do its own thing. Once our sex center returns to its innocent and natural state, it has been purified and "deconditioned." The sexual energy is no longer compressed outward in release, but begins to turn, impressing itself inward and upward. The sense is one of the sex center now being free of a force or restriction that was holding it down. Once free, sexual energy knows no rules, no limitations. The bodies choose the style according to the level of presence and sexual energy available. Sometimes it's still and serene and the next moment out of the core of this stillness, there is expansive movement. Each stroke, each thrust, each penetration received in its own right, complete relaxation. Wild and passionate going absolutely nowhere.

True passion is a glorious celebration of the body where everything is incorporated in the present moment. It means to be wild but not unconscious in it, and then wildness is beautiful. True wildness has no direction, no goal, it's simply here and here and here! Divisions disappear as bodies slip out of time and move into orgasmic unity through presence.

KEY POINTS:

୧≈ There's more to sex than orgasm and ejaculation.

୧≈ A man's ejaculation of semen is not true orgasm.

୧≈ A woman's orgasmic potential expands with receptivity not tension.

୧≈ The energy of desire can be inverted to thrilling effect.

୧≈ Forget about orgasm and become orgasmic through relaxation.

19

NON-EJACULATION

ONE OF THE CONFUSIONS about ejaculation is that it is valued as a form of relaxation. But it is really a dissipation, a tremendous loss of energy which results in fatigue or irritation rather than the refreshing quality typical of relaxation. Ancient Taoist principles whereby a man derives good health through living in harmony with the universe, embraced the phenomenon of non-ejaculation, retaining the semen in the body, and reabsorbing the life force into longevity.

Likewise, Tantra is interested in non-ejaculation which is not to be confused with ejaculation *control*. Non-ejaculation means that the question of ejaculation rarely enters the picture. It is not even an issue, because you are relaxing into it. This enables lovemaking to be a prolonged and satisfying exchange. On the other hand, to *control* your ejaculation implies that a strong urge to ejaculate is present, and it needs repressing. It then becomes an act of sheer will where the sex energy is first intentionally built up to a peak; and then mental control is exerted to retract from ejaculation. A woman then finds herself at the mercy of her partner when he cries out, "Stop! Don't move!" This is devastating to say the least, when all she needed was that one last stroke to come!

Many techniques exist today mistakenly in the name of Tantra, which are based on this idea of repeatedly controlling ejaculation, of dancing on the verge, of playing with the fire.

But the results are less than pleasing as men complain of feelings of congestion and aches and pains in the groin or testicles. It happens because the whole system is geared up for release, and then stops, perhaps several times, as the energy is switched on and off, on and off. While this dancing with danger may give an immediate pleasure and high, or a feeling of vitality, frequently there is a corresponding low some time later. A congested residue of tension in the genital and belly area remains and as a style of lovemaking, eventually it may put stress on the prostate gland, causing discomfort and physical problems.

The very word "control" implies a tension, so ejaculation control cannot be a relaxing experience. The tension of the urgent ejaculation *and* the tension of controlling it with the mind create a double tension. The delights of Tantric lovemaking arise from a relaxing *into* the sex energy, a state of acceptance where nothing is forced. It focuses on an unhurried, gentle expansion of the sexual energy through relaxation and sensuality, and excitement and tension are not part of this picture. The genitals through their own intelligence, the positive and negative polarities, challenge each other, which creates a natural sexual ecstasy. The sex organs begin to operate beneath excitement. And nothing is fixed beforehand, nothing is guaranteed. Some days it is electrical or totally riveting in intensity, and other days there is a timeless or floating quality. In this kind of experience, ejaculation seems light years away.

Orgasm and the ego

Unfortunately, both men and women have been programmed to identify their partner's orgasm as pleasure that they themselves have been responsible for creating. And a man, particularly, feels that a woman's orgasms prove him to be more of a man, strengthening his sexual ego. But when he keeps a woman revolving around the superficial layer of her sexual energy by insisting that she come in order to satisfy himself, he limits his own sexual potential. The doorway to great transformation remains closed.

Conversely, women really like their man to ejaculate even if they themselves do not manage to come. I have heard them say that they feel cheated if the man does not ejaculate, feeling that he is holding something back from them. Or, most common, they use it to finish off the sex act, since every woman knows exactly how to make her man ejaculate. This attitude reflects the woman's desire to control her man, to encourage him to lose his life-giving semen, and thereby his authority. It is her conditioning to try to run the show in her ignorance of her divine feminine power. The truth is with the man becoming less identified with ejaculation, with it becoming less important to him, then the woman has a long-awaited opportunity to begin to make love with feminine receptivity and within her polarity. She is by nature relaxed and graceful, and she discovers a new sexual world far more pleasurable than that of hunting an orgasm. When she is authentic, she becomes orgasmic and glowing, the source of love. This can change her life and the life of her partner too.

Naturally, the desire to ejaculate will come and go while you make love, but a desire is different from an overwhelming urge. Desire is still an idea in the mind, and the urge is a need of the body. If you are in that twilight zone where you are unable to relax during lovemaking because of a powerful or persistent urge to ejaculate, *please* allow it to happen. Ejaculate and remain present in your ejaculation. Enjoy it, feeling every moment. Tantra suggests that when a man is struggling with himself, trying to keep his urges under control, it is healthier to ejaculate, because fighting it will also cause a double tension. This tension is likely to persist as restlessness after making love and will appear again next time, creating a cycle of tension. Tantra encourages relaxation in both mind and body, so if the man must ejaculate, it is best to just do it. Then he will soon be able to start anew.

As a man develops a new way of sensing his penis, at times he is likely to experience intense, unadulterated pleasure especially during deep, sustained penetration. As the vaginal walls are being awakened with love and consciousness, the intensity of the experience is so overwhelming that it almost reminds him of excitement and the temptation to move with it and go for it will arise. However, men have found that if they really feel into the penis, beneath this veneer of excitement the sensations are of a distinctly different quality, the source of tremendous satisfaction as the male positive energy starts to move through the woman for the first time. So when the temptations of ejaculation appear it is often well worth it to remain relaxed and keep it to a non-ejaculation.

How do you feel afterward?

As you begin to experiment with and without orgasm and ejaculation, be guided by how you feel in the minutes and hours afterward. As I began to experiment with orgasm and my lover's ejaculation, sometimes going for it, sometimes not, I began to observe how I felt afterward and not during, but later, even much later. This provided valuable information, and I discovered that I experienced greater well-being when I had not forced an orgasm, when apparently nothing had happened. For men too, these questions are a valuable guideline: "How do you feel when you do?" and "How do you feel when you don't?" Your experience will give you all the answers. It is your most significant teacher.

KEY POINTS:

ॐ As a man relaxes, the powerful urge for ejaculation decreases gradually.

ॐ Non-ejaculation is not to be confused with ejaculation control.

ॐ The first implies relaxation, and the other tension.

ॐ Controlling the urge for ejaculation suppresses the energy with possible congesting effects.

ॐ Non-ejaculation increases vitality and creativity.

20

PREMATURE EJACULATION

PREMATURE EJACULATION is normally defined as ejaculation prior to mutual satisfaction. This can be as simple as immediate ejaculation upon penetration or unexpected, uncontrollable ejaculation. It could be ten, fifteen, even twenty minutes—the exact time period differs for everyone. It ends the sex act, finished or not. There is inadequate time for sexual maturity, in a way. Countless men suffer in unspeakable isolation the anguish of premature ejaculation, and yet it is an extremely common phenomenon. It is important for men to realize that it is more of a psychological problem. The repressions of sex, the tensions surrounding it, the lack of information, are the underlying problems here, not the body itself. These tensions and anxieties affect the mind of a man creating a substantial amount of presexual excitement. When the situation finally presents itself, the internal stresses, pressures, and anxieties are so great, the sexual excitement so overwhelming, that the man ejaculates uncontrollably.

To understand when and how this happens, think for a moment about the basic concept of polarity. The positive energy of the man flows out of the penis and is received by the woman into the vagina, the negative pole. Because the woman has been relying on movement and clitoral stimulation for her sexual experience, a disturbance has built up in her vagina making it expectant and demanding. Remember too, there are the tensions from our collective past that lie hidden from consciousness. When we add excitement and titillation during foreplay, the disturbance reflects as tension and tightness in the vaginal walls, creating a kind of craving, a hunger. Sometimes this can become so intense it is actually painful, and the whole area feels like it is getting narrow and contracted. And so when penetration occurs, the woman is not receptive but also full up, almost defensive, and the circuit for the energy flow is interrupted.

Understanding sexual excitement

The man (naturally a positive charge), with his own social tensions and excitement, and now overly positive, enters the disturbed vaginal environment of the woman. Here he meets unexpectedly another excited or disturbed charge. Now the energy of the male has nowhere to go, no way of flowing into the vagina. It has to go somewhere, so it meets the resistance, and explodes overflowing into ejaculation prematurely.

It is essential to understand how the woman contributes to premature ejaculation too, either inadvertently or consciously. At any time during intercourse a sexual image or intense stimulation can trigger this excitable charge to move in the woman, causing the energy to rush down in a wave of excitement, resulting in the man's sudden and unexpected ejaculation, as though almost pulled from him. Or intentionally, a woman is capable of creating enough sexual tension in her vagina at any time to forcefully have sex completed. Of course there are repercussions, as this kind of action severs the potential thread to her femininity.

As the man penetrates the woman, the state of the vagina gives the penis immediate information on how to behave. If the vagina is excited, it will be tight and defensive, making the man restless and tense and more likely to come. If it is relaxed and calm, silky and embracing, the penis responds to this invitation with a thrilling life force, positive flowing into negative. The importance of understanding sexual excitement cannot be overemphasized. Once you begin to develop the capacity to identify it as and when it appears, then you are no longer held in its unconscious grip. Instead you can play with it in order to best suit your needs, and shed some light and understanding where there has previously been compulsion or confusion.

The main guideline to avoid premature ejaculation is straight-forward. Men and women should not build up a great deal of excitement before making love. Starting with soft penetration is also advised. When two people remove the internal pressures and expectations of sex, fear is reduced and so too, is the tension. It also helps to make a date to make love, because it reduces one major source of anxiety for the man knowing he *will* make love. There is less apprehension or uncertainty when he knows that he need not persuade the woman. It is precisely these kinds of tensions, fears, and preoccupations that contribute to over-excitement and the event of premature ejaculation. Where there is no persuasion, when we don't have to tempt and turn each other on, we can enter lovemaking consciously, in a more relaxed frame of mind, and gradually our disturbing patterns of the past dissolve. Where there is no anxiety, gradually the lovemaking can be extended to last for hours.

Stay relaxed and speak to each other

As suggested during a fresh look at foreplay, you both need to stay as relaxed as possible, focusing on simple contact, sensuality, and touch. Touch the breasts and genitals in a way that acknowledges them and warmly says hello, rather than stimulating them. Awaken rather than excite, and from this relaxed state sexual arousal will emerge naturally and beautifully. As soon as sexual response occurs, penetrate. Tell her you are erect. Ask the woman if she is ready. As soon as you are ready, tell the man you want him inside you now. It helps so much to cooperate in this way, instead of each person doing his or her own guesswork. Don't wait until you are both really excited; it's better to penetrate well before that. Through this lack of excitement the genitals remain cool and ejaculation is less likely. Penetrate as soon as it is appropriate so that you avoid remaining in the pre-stages of lovemaking for too long. And make the first penetration as slow as possible, having eye contact with each other so as to keep you present. For a man it is advised to keep his awareness on and in his penis, and not to think about where he is putting it. When he thinks about the vagina, he is flooded with all his mental associations with sex, his sexual fantasies, which again encourage ejaculation.

Some men notice that they ejaculate quite easily with one woman, and yet with someone else they maintain an erection for a long time without ejaculation. This is confusing, and many men will have wondered why. More often than not it has to do with the woman herself, and not the man. It depends a great deal on the environment in which the penis finds itself. If a woman is relaxed and disinterested in excitement or orgasm, the vagina is serene, warm, and calm, and lovemaking can be prolonged for hours. When a woman tends toward excitability, premature ejaculation is highly possible.

As you can see, women contribute enormously to a man's tendency to ejaculate prematurely, so it is really worthwhile if you don't make your man too excited. Then a man is a more potent lover, and a woman is fully satisfied. So much more is to be gained if we try relaxing into the sexual energy instead of activating it. Unfortunately, the woman's conditioning has taught her that moving and stimulating the clitoris, getting agitated and active, and hunting for an orgasm is what lovemaking is all about. She thinks that this is what the man is looking for, too. The thought of relaxing into the more feminine, receptive dimension of sexual experience seems to contradict her ideas of enjoyment. But when we learn to cool down in sex, and so enable the man to be cool too, the doorway to ecstasy begins to ease open.

In order to create the possibility of longer-lasting sexual union, allow the man inside your vagina as soon as possible so his anticipation does not build up. When you feel mentally and physically prepared for penetration, invite it. Communicate. Ask him to penetrate you. Let the first penetration be especially slow, and once he is inside, keep relaxing the vaginal muscles imagining them to be soft and welcoming. Don't move unnecessarily. Be more physically passive and receptive (this does not mean dead or laidback, but less outgoing, and more physically present, responsive rather than demonstrative) and let the focus be within your body and what is happening there—the whole glorious phenomenon of it. This inward glance is worth far more than the effects of repeated pelvic movements, and it will surprise you. When your consciousness enters the atmosphere, relaxation and sensuality flood through your bodies. Take your time, don't force anything, don't hurry, don't try to inflame the energy. Just turn on enough, penetrate and be penetrated, and then stay with this initial attraction, keeping yourself in the present, rooting yourself in the body, using any of the Love Keys.

KEY POINTS:

క The cause of premature ejaculation lies in sexual tension and anxiety.

క Reduce sexual anticipation and excitement prior to penetration.

క A woman unknowingly contributes to premature ejaculation.

క Introducing a conscious relaxed approach can eliminate this problem.

21

ERECTION AND IMPOTENCE

S OME MEN HAVE DIFFICULTIES with erection; others don't. Some need a few attempts before they can manage an erection and others get an erection by just thinking about it. Some can have an erection easily with one woman, and with another they cannot. It can be a confusing, misunderstood phenomenon, and the source of much pain and torment for men *and* women.

The most damaging part of this confusion is that many men, if nor all, estimate their manliness according to their capacity to be erect and satisfy a woman. Women often estimate men in the same way. How hard can he get and how long can he hold it hard? All of this operates as an enormous burden for a man; it eats away at him while his mind casts self-doubt on his capacity to love a woman, he even begins to doubt her. His psychology begins to invade the naturalness and integrity of his sexual expression. Slowly an immense pressure and tension builds up in him but, ironically, the truth is that a woman is also responsible for a man's erection.

The power of sexual magnetism without excitement

If we begin to look at the penis and vagina as a unit,

counterparts of one whole with magnetic intelligence, our understanding of sex can begin to shift. Instead of a mental pressure slowly accumulating in the man, which dictates that in order to make love he must do something, he would be more accurate in considering his penis to be an instrument of love that *responds* to the love in his counterpart, the vagina. This means he does not force an erection by doing something, but trusts love and waits until an erection swells and grows either inside or outside the vagina. When the vagina is instilled with consciousness and love, erection happens very easily and with no effort at all. The penis seeks out the vaginal depths with astonishing alacrity. Women know how to be sexy or provocative to help a man get hard, and it is something they do willingly so that sex happens. But when the focus is outward, directed on the man and not inward on herself, her attempts will frequently be futile. When a woman tries to stimulate the man into erection with her hand or mouth, for instance, she is overlooking an important fact. It is her vagina, this nuclear part of her, which makes or breaks an erection, and man is only half of this miraculous phenomenon. The welcoming liquid quality of the vaginal cavity with its embracing velveteen silkiness is what will do the job.

Men who have experienced both styles of lovemaking, excitement versus relaxation, say that it is possible to feel the difference between a potent erection and an excitable one. The first, they report, feels elastic and easy and sensitive, while the second feels brittle, hard, and yet easy to lose. It is like the difference between the vibrancy of a snake and the deadness of a stick. I recall a man who had been experimenting with the Love Keys sharing his astute observation, "I get two different kinds of erections. One way, I move into relaxation and non-doing, and after a while a movement of energy happens and an erection is there. This kind of erection does not go soft when there is no movement. The other way, I move into excitement and tension and I get an erection that feels hollow because it is not connected with my insides. I lose this kind of erection if there is no movement." Many men will have experienced the same phenomenon.

Another man in one of my workshops said, "When I consciously push an erection by tightening the perineum and the anal area, the energy becomes concentrated in my pelvis. In contrast, when I remain relaxed and conscious of my entire pelvic area, the energy falls back naturally and the perineum does its own thing. It still feels the same, which was confusing at first. But when I let it happen, it is like I am available to it, rather than forcing it. I can feel a contracting sensation in the perineum and the root of my penis pushing upward, more like squeezing than spasms. This feeling is absolutely wonderful and at the same time relaxed because I am making no effort. It's just happening."

Experience an electrical surge of inspiration

The design of the sex organs, the penis fitting so well inside the vagina as it does, enables the energy to flow naturally and erection is a by product of the attraction. Erection can also happen close to the vagina, not necessarily inside. The natural probing and forward thrusting of the penis when it comes into the vaginal presence is the positive energy seeking its complementary counterpart, in order to experience completion. This polarization of the penis where it responds through polarity has been described by men as a journey from the head of the penis to the root of the penis. The entire penis becomes potent and this expands the magnetic phenomenon. When the man can imagine his penis emerging from the root of his body as a shaft of consciousness, or a stream of light, he becomes increasingly aware of its entire length, sensing aliveness through it fully.

The penis is *extremely* sensitive to shifts in environment. It feels when the vagina is present and relaxed, and when it is not. It knows when the vagina is moving out of polarity, for example when the woman begins to make efforts to achieve orgasm. When the open, relaxed surroundings of the vagina become narrow and constricted from a receptive attitude to a demanding one, the man will often experience an immediate loss of erection. The sensitivity of a conscious penis cannot meet such a demand and will shrink away as the erection diminishes, or while fully erect he may even flop out sideways in sudden disinterest.

When the penis is lying erect inside the woman, the man will usually begin to lose his erection at the precise moment when the consciousness of the woman leaves her vagina. The penis is *that* sensitive. This loss of erection can be due to a single thought. It has shocked me time and again how the second I allow my awareness to drift away, the penis will instantly shrink. It makes sense; its electrical counterpart has gone away, absented itself. When I am able to reconnect with my body, immerse myself in it again and quit thinking, the penis will stretch out and snake up slowly into the vagina once again, regaining lost ground.

The penis is especially sensitive to the energy in the breasts, a phenomenon that both man and woman are able to feel. When the breasts are activated the penis responds instantly. This is because the vagina becomes receptive and sensitive when breasts become filled with life, more positive. This in turn enables the man's energy to be drawn from the penis into the vagina. The woman, while focusing on her breasts and receiving the man, will feel the penis suddenly respond with added life as the electricity moves within. This intensification of polarity, even if created for only a few moments, will be experienced by the penis as a jolt of energy, a surge of fire, an inspiration. When the breasts are truly open and loving from within, a woman will feel that she is penetrating a man with love through her breasts, chest, and heart, activating his heart and love in turn.

This shows us that the life in the penis depends on the life within the vagina, that the greater the capacity of both men and women to be present and conscious during lovemaking, the greater the ecstasy they will experience. If it feels a bit dead while you are making love, this can be an indication that you are not really here. You may be tired or preoccupied perhaps, but not really with your lover in the spirit of love. The more you become practiced at stepping into "here" the more alive the genitals will be to each other.

Psychology and impotence

Impotence is man's greatest fear. It is a shock to a man when his penis does not or will not rise to the occasion, when no amount of stimulation or excitement will do it, and in time videos, skimpy clothing or sexy devices will not help either. This can often astound a man who in earlier years was known as a stud. But this is where impotence will most commonly occur. The trouble is that the penis has become insensitive and unresponsive due to an over-dependence on excitement, and if a man has not explored his sexuality from within, impotence easily prevails. He has sadly become immune to his sexual energy, self-doubt creeps in, frustration and anger grow. Millions of men today suffer from impotence, a problem as chronic as premature ejaculation.

Impotence is frequently blamed on the partner, on the familiarity of years spent together, the routine of old habits, the layers of emotional barriers and the pain of unspoken wounds that lie across the heart. The love that initially joined two people all those years ago has become inaccessible, and there is a loss of stimulus and attraction. We have also come to believe that older men need to be invigorated, abandoning their wives for younger women. But the problem of impotence lies not with the partner, but with the insensitivity of the penis and with the psychology of the man himself.

When sex just doesn't work anymore

In the case of impotence, Tantra tells us the penis is no longer functioning as an authentic positive male pole; it has become flaccid and unresponsive, having lost its innate interest and sensitivity. It is no longer rooted in the unlimited pool of sexual energy. Instead, the cumulative years of sexual misunderstanding and misuse have made the genitals insensitive and numb. Sensation took over from sensitivity a long time ago, and men have never been taught how the penis genuinely works inside the vagina, how to develop the inherent magnetic properties to give them and their partners lasting love and satisfaction.

For an impotent man there are no options; he has no access to his ecstasy while his pleasure has been reduced to occasional moments of release, superficial and fleeting. His capacity to be erect, mostly a function of his mind, his sexual imagination and fantasies, has atrophied. His experience of sensation is what he *imagines* is happening to him, instead of what is *actually* happening.

These days it is socially accepted to claim that sex just doesn't work anymore. Sex is cast aside, seemingly unimportant, but the lack of a willing expressive sexual energy soon becomes the source of self-doubt and is the underlying cause of disagreements and emotional discontent between couples. When a man is without sexual expression, he will soon feel the corrosive effects of his stagnant energy and will become restless, bored, critical, easy to displease and quick to anger. When men compensate by channeling their sexual energy into work and achievement, leaving no time for love, a pivotal part of them remains unexpressed and undernourished. Later, surrounded by material wealth, they wonder at their unhappiness, their problems of obesity, alcoholism, and impotence. As important as they thought money was, suddenly they see that their priorities have been misplaced.

Overcoming lack of feeling together

According to Tantra, both men and women are responsible for male impotence. After years of friction-oriented lovemaking, the genitals, both male and female, have grown increasingly insensitive, the muscle tissues becoming hard and tight. When the penis lies without movement in the vagina, there will be no tingling, vibrating, or sensitivity, no subtle awareness. After years of gross contact, the penis may possibly become erect only if there is friction; and without it, there are no feelings, no delicate sensations, no innate vitality. The erection response through polarity effect is deadened and inaccessible, a disturbance in the bio-energy. Fortunately couples can overcome the problem of impotence together. It requires patience, sensitivity, and self-respect. Respect yourself, respect your energy, respect your genitals and give them time to heal and balance. Make a date to make love frequently. Give yourselves plenty of time, exchange massage of breasts, penis, and testicles. Be unhurried and conscious, relax together. When you are both ready, lie in bed and try penetration without erection. (described in chapter 12 on Soft Penetration). Once successfully inserted, and even the head is enough, maintain the consciousness in the penis and vagina, exchange energy through eye contact. A woman must remember to hold awareness in the breasts too, and a man must intensify her awareness by touching them. Try this way of making love again and again and it will happen that from this neutral place, erection will arise *in response to the vagina*. Even if only for a short time at first, it will give you an inspiring insight into the wonderful phenomenon of erection, and the way out of impotence. Stop looking for immediate gratification or results because it may take many attempts before the positive and negative begin to respond and operate according to design. But when a man can start relaxing into the ambience of love with his partner and begin to trust his penis then the natural intelligence of the sex organs can be re-established. Erection will once more become a natural response.

Disastrously, science has produced an "impotence pill" with an astonishing effect—a man requires the usual sexual stimulus or provocation (so it is not an aphrodisiac) whereupon full erection follows! In the short term this does offer consolation, but in the context of male polarity lying at the source of man's erectile capacity, the glaring truth is that medical intervention exacerbates an already dire situation and offers no insight into the energetic realities involved. The man is already chronically insensitive and unaware of himself, and this finally turns him into an erection machine, intensifying his insensitivity to himself and of course his woman. Even while she may be very grateful to experience penetration once again, the dullness in the penis does not allow for the awakening of her ecstatic sexual energies. Neither does it generate love.

Insensitivity resulting from tension and anxiety

I hear sometimes from men about a "sexual condition" which is an extreme erectile function but with virtually no sexual sensitivity. This means an erection can be maintained for prolonged periods, but the penis is so insensitive that it is impossible to build up enough sensation to trigger an ejaculation. And so they pump away incessantly and end up frustrated in the absence of a few seconds of real pleasure. This in a sense can also be classified as impotence, even while it appears to be the opposite. When a man has an erection that is steel hard but without consciousness in it, he is effectively impotent. Where he has no sense of his male pole responding to a woman, he feels less manly. A friend of mine who experienced excruciating emotional pain about his insensitivity from his early sexual years was fortunate enough to meet a woman twenty years later who was interested in experimenting with him. After a period of eight months of making love without the tensions and anxieties that produced his insensitivity, he was grateful to find his penis beginning to regain its inherent sensitivity, able to sense the environment surrounding it and respond accordingly. He began to experience his penis as a channel of divine energy, able to sustain love and deeply awaken the woman within. The organic intelligence present in the body is a force so powerfully integrating that even the slightest shift in consciousness (which reduces the pressure of our sexual conditioning) is rewarded by the vigor of renewed life and sensitivity. The body is intrinsically ready (even longing) to return to one organic unity.

KEY POINTS:

ह~ Erection is not a mechanical function but a polarity response to the woman.

ह~ The woman influences erection through consciousness in the vagina and breasts.

ह~Erection is the natural outcome in the presence of consciousness and love.

ह~Impotence reflects the man's extreme insensitivity to himself and to his partner.

ह~Soft penetration is very helpful in restoring a man's trust and sensitivity in his penis.

22

FEELINGS AND EMOTIONS

TANTRA IS A JOURNEY from mind to body, from thinking to feeling. As we immerse ourselves in the world of feeling, we will become aware that there are two distinct categories. There are feelings that have an emotional content such as sadness or irritation, or those that are the sensations of energy movement within the body itself. As couples practice using the Love Keys, they will discover both kinds of feelings. While gradually increasing their consciousness in lovemaking, they will find a corresponding increase in bodily sensitivity and awareness. This brings in a whole new range of internal sensations and feelings such as smoothness, velvet silkiness, heat and warmth, excitation, tingling, bubbling, lightness, fluffiness, coolness, molten gold, streaming brilliancy, and dissolution of all physical boundaries. As we reduce the need for sensation in sex, we uncover in ourselves an innate sensitivity and perceive a world of unknown sensations lying within. This gives sexual delight as the energy begins to move along internal circuits. The sexual experience becomes entirely different and at first couples do not describe it as exactly sexual in nature. In a recent workshop of mine, after his first taste of it, one man said "It is really touching, and it is not like anything you see in the movies!"

Our feelings are different from our emotions

Feelings that have an emotional content are another matter entirely, and confuse many people because they can seem to create heaven and hell. Argument and love get entangled again and again, and there seems to be no way through to the peaceful times. Our feelings and emotions keep disturbing the tranquillity. It is this aspect of ourselves, this subtle and usually unconscious layer, that needs to be brought into the awareness. Awareness of the body and of the thoughts are the first two steps. This is relatively easy compared to the third step, awareness of our shifting moods, swings in temperament, and complex emotions.

Although the words "emotion" and "feeling" are used interchangeably, this is a common mistake. There is a vast difference between the experience of an emotion and the experience of a feeling. This distinction is important to understand, particularly in the world of love, since it offers insights into our psychology and gives us the possible start to taking real responsibility for ourselves. Knowing the difference enables you to know what is happening, when it is happening.

Feelings are an expression of what is happening now, consciously in the present moment, and emotions are an unconscious expression from the past, something that has already happened. Feelings are conscious while emotions operate on an unconscious level. Feelings are expressed freshly and innocently, while with emotion the expression is avoided, repressed, or delayed, and when finally expressed is often overwhelming, destructive, or unkind. Emotions like to blame and say "you always... it is your fault. . . while feelings take responsibility and say "I feel" or "I need". Feelings strengthen the heart while emotions harden the ego. Feelings bring you closer to the one you love while emotions separate you. It is clear that feelings and emotions have very different qualities, and give us almost opposing experiences of reality. Through our feelings we expand our energy, we feel light and energized. We feel closer to the one we love and supported by life. Through emotions we are contracted and tense, experiencing heaviness, hopelessness, and pain. It is exhausting. We feel separated from the world and outcast by the one we love.

How ignored feelings become emotional monsters

In our society, where rationality and reason are given prime status, our feelings, whatever they may be, are given almost no importance by ourselves or others. Unfortunately, in most cases we try to repress them in order to reveal less about our vulnerabilities and weaknesses. Ignoring our true feelings begins in early childhood, when we learn to hold ourselves together. This is true especially of men and feelings are regarded as belonging strictly to the female domain. The English expression "keeping a stiff upper lip" is no joke because when we are in touch with our feelings, our insecurities, and weaknesses, the upper lip and chin will tremble shamelessly. When any feelings of sadness or frustration, even joy and love remain unexpressed, they accumulate slowly and become a storehouse of emotions affecting the harmony of mind and body. Jealousy, anger, hatred, fear, and rage, start building up early in our lives (often related to sexual interference), and no matter how hard we repress them, it is not easy to ignore these past emotions in the body. Our social lack of honest expression has compelled us to develop tough, brittle, and defensive qualities. We store the pain and disappointments that would have us weep and wail, and so they bury themselves in the unconscious as emotions, distorting our bodies and damaging the psyche.

These unexpressed feelings live on in us and return sooner or later as destructive emotions. The ghosts of the past continually taint the simplicity of the present. This explains why a seemingly placid and reasonable person can one day erupt at the slightest provocation, exploding irrationally into a violent rage. They are releasing the pent-up pressure of past feelings that can no longer be suppressed, and the virulence of such an outburst is rarely proportional to the incident that set it off. The accumulation of stored and unexpressed feelings is released with the force of this pressure behind it, so it seems to make the person act completely "unreasonably," but in reality they are acting "unconsciously." If we can become aware of the influence of our past on our present moment we can begin to separate emotions and real feelings.

Expressing our feelings as we experience them

Feelings, on other hand, are consciously expressed at the time when the feeling is actually happening. It is not stored or repressed, but exposed. If anger is present, or frustration, a wholesome roar from the belly for several seconds can have a truly liberating effect. The anger dissolves instantly, and there is no lingering resentment gnawing away at you. Conversely, you are exhilarated and full of heart-pounding life. When it is an aching, breaking heart, an animal-like wail of crying pain will make the whole thing more bearable. The internal pressure is released. Sadness is expressed in heartfelt tears. When we show our innermost feelings as we experience them happening within us, they are transformed into living energy and we are freed from any undermining effects. Even unexpressed love or joy soon turns to depression or sadness.

The point is that our conscious feelings contain our heaven, while our unconscious emotions contain our hell, and we create our hell through not expressing our heaven. Emotion is a defense to pain while feeling embraces it and uses it as a way to heal. At times heaven may look like hell in the form of a tragedy, a loss or a disaster, but if we allow the *real* feelings to rise, the anguish, agony and pain, we feel much better, even uplifted. Otherwise, if unexpressed our feelings pull down the spirit and eat up the heart. These remain as emotions lying dormant in the unconscious until an incident triggers the memory. The best we can do is to learn to share our feelings and so avoid our emotions.

Storing feelings in the body

The body functions as an innocent "home" for these unexpressed feelings. This creates an internal pressure, the stress of which can go so far as to affect one's physical structure and muscular movement. When feeling is unexpressed, the body stores it in the tissues. The way a person angles their jaw and holds their head, uses their shoulders, carries their pelvis, are all determined by internal emotional pressure. When the sexual center is contorted through the tension of our emotions as it is in all of us, this too, is evident in the walk, the angle of the pelvis, the shape of the legs, the alignment through the knees. It is in the solar plexus, however, where many of our unreleased emotions are stored, damaging physical and energetic structure.

When we are emotional and observant of the solar plexus, we will notice the discomforting gnawing sensation of being ill at ease, even a ceaseless twisting and turning. Awareness and relaxation of the solar plexus while making love is suggested earlier as a Love Key because it intensifies presence and sexual energy. In the same way, the solar plexus can be used in daily life as a monitor of the emotions. It gives great insight. As soon as you observe that there is a physical feeling, a hooking or pulling in the solar plexus, know that ease has been disturbed, and something is afoot. You are emotional! The solar plexus never misreads the situation, and it does not have to be a particularly dramatic event. It could be something as mild as a friend ignoring you in the coffee shop, a neighbor saying something dismissive about your children or your dog, or your preoccupied partner forgetting to give you a good-bye kiss. You may notice later that you feel disturbed, especially in the stomach area, with a feeling of separation or unhappiness.

Awareness, acceptance, and relief of tension

Instead of carrying around the discomfort of this emotion all day, acknowledge to yourself precisely what you are feeling— abandoned or insecure and simply feel it, experiencing the physical aspect of the feeling too. Enter into the solar plexus with your awareness and sink down into the feeling there. Remain with it for a while, imagining flames in the base of your belly burning it up. After some time check to see how you are feeling. How is your sense of ease? Having acknowledged your emotion by bringing awareness to its root, you are likely to have experienced some relief, a lightness of spirit. The physical load is dissolved, the acceptance of it dispels the tension, and you are rooted in your being again. In this case there is nothing more to be done, and you are able to continue your day with a joyful heart.

You may, however, need to call your partner and tell him you miss him, or to speak to your friend, find out how they are and share your feelings with them. You may discover too, that they did not even see you in the coffee shop, engrossed as they were in their own morning blues. Suddenly, the whole scenario disappears in a puff of smoke. In reality it was your personal insecurity, the need to be acknowledged and valued, that was offended. And this triggered the emotions always simmering within. If you find that acknowledging the emotion is not adequate in itself, you may need to do more to release the discomfort. Always try something physical for some minutes, jumping up and down, stamping your feet on the ground, or beating a pillow with your fists, even chattering away in gibberish aloud to yourself. All movement and sound helps tremendously to reduce the undermining effect of emotions in the body.

With a little more intense awareness we can start reflecting on our emotions, moods, our momentary ups and downs. This requires real alertness, and is difficult because the emotions are effectively a layer in the body. We experience them as an integral aspect of ourselves, we think it is who we are. Maintaining awareness of the solar plexus is of great assistance in detecting subtle emotions, and it is important to dissolve the accompanying tensions in the solar plexus through the awareness. Otherwise they accumulate and penetrate our psyche. The expression of an emotion is always beneficial because it removes internal pressures from the system. However, it is the *awareness of the emotion* not the emotion itself, which begins to dissolve the threads that link us to our unconscious aspects. Through this observation, the emotions gradually cease to be motivated. The past remains in the past. When feelings arise in the present they are then uncontaminated by incomplete experiences from the past and can be expressed in their freshness and purity. As this happens, love and life begin to take on a childlike simplicity.

Love, emotion, and sexual healing

When we begin the sexual act, we do so with the tension of all our unexpressed feelings, the now fragile emotions within us. In the sexual arena our emotions get activated unsuspectingly and come into play, casting shadows on our lives without our knowing it. This has disastrous results in love, and we find ourselves repeatedly in the same argument or dissatisfaction with our lover as if we are going around in circles. Or the same issue will separate you from a series of partners you have loved and left, because the theme keeps replaying itself. We can't seem to get it right. Yet, in our ignorance of what love really is, we have come to accept the ups and downs to be an essential part of love. When we become conscious of the effects and particularly the roots of our emotions in the past, we can begin to take more responsibility for our love and separate it from the emotional area. We can start to create it afresh, bringing intelligence and awareness into the act of love and to express our feelings as we stop identifying with our emotions.

Although it shows up differently in men and women, the genitals of both sexes are loaded with shame and accumulated negative emotions that interfere with the natural polarity. Once we take the pressure off the penis and vagina by removing the driving need to do something in sex, the genital poles will start a process of relaxation. As they do so, the encapsulated emotions will begin to be released in different ways. A man should not be embarrassed to cry and show his feelings, and indeed his task is to be as honest and straight as he can be. Your partner will thank you and be grateful for sharing your vulnerability, especially since in the moment of releasing tears you will feel the penis more sensitive and conscious. A male friend of mine, as a boy in puberty, noticed some marks developing on his penis. He was utterly distressed, thinking there was something wrong with him. He could not talk to anyone about it. And because he had never seen a penis before other than his own, he was not to know the markings were entirely normal. He wanted to see a doctor, but this meant discussing the matter with his parents first, which was inconceivable. Instead he buried his shame and mortification and well into his late thirties he unconsciously felt his penis to be "sick." Only when he began to make love consciously did this shame and pain emerge from his body. When it did, he realized how these emotions had affected all his sexual encounters with women. Allowing yourself to feel again what you failed to feel years before is a healing in itself, which extends to the genital tissue. With the onslaught of tears which help to wash away pain and to free the body of internal stresses and toxins, a new sensitivity arises in the sex organs. The poles slowly empty out, losing their disturbances (negative consciousness) and regaining their true polarity. In this way the man becomes more masculine, the woman more feminine.

How the past can disturb the present

In my work with people it has been very distressing to discover that a high percentage of women have been sexually abused, many as very young girls. This is surprisingly common in men too, although to a lesser degree. Such individuals retain the pain and confusion of shocking early sexual events into their adulthood. Invariably they were unable to tell anyone, to share or express their feelings of fear and horror. Perhaps it involved father, grandfather, uncle, brother, or the next-door neighbor, or even the local priest. Mothers have been known to accuse their own daughters of being sexually provocative, blaming the child rather than believing a report of sexual molestation. These powerful imprints live in the body and the mind, underlying all future encounters. Years after the events, withheld feelings have become emotions that can rise to the surface and seek release in an attempt to be free of the secretive, shadowy past.

The basis of the sexually healing experience is the resurfacing and releasing of past feelings, rage, pain, and frustrations, the remnants of which have left an imprint in the sex organs. The relaxation that we are after can and will cause painful memories to resurface in an attempt to remove the obstructing tensions in an otherwise freely flowing energy system. With this understanding we can welcome old childhood wounds and stored negative experiences that start to emerge as the genitals increase in consciousness and begin their healing process. When my own pain was triggered, I shed tears that were achingly deep, at times with strong and uncontrollable contorting body movements, shaking, shivering, and perspiring. To this day, I don't know what specific incidents created the pain, but I found that the release, not the origin was significant. Through releasing long-withheld feelings, a melting sensation and sweetness arose in my vagina and healing took place.

I have always maintained that the bed is not the place for analysis; this is love, not therapy. For me it was best not to speak about it or try and explain what was happening, but rather to continue making love while the tears were flowing, to keep opening myself to the penis triggering these past feelings in me. If I pulled away and rolled into a collapsed heap, or tried to talk about it, my tears would dry up immediately and I would be left feeling flat or incomplete. If I stayed present in my lovemaking, facing my lover and the intensity of what I was feeling, breathing deeply and allowing the vulnerability and tears, I would access a deeper layer of withheld emotions. As each layer peeled away I found more feeling and perception in my vagina, and my lover felt his penis respond too.

Noticing emotion as it arises

It is important to recognize when the past and unconsciousness step in, and when *precisely* emotion knocks on your door. How you deal with it makes all the difference. For instance, while you are making love, a rough, insensitive touch by your lover could remind you of an unloving uncle who did the same thing to you when you were a little girl, and an old emotion gets triggered. Even the smallest movement can be telling. Suddenly, the confusion and apprehension of the childhood experience can flood through you, bringing feelings of repulsion, curiosity, fear, guilt, attraction, or pain. The past has placed its ugly scarring foot into the beauty of your present love, and suddenly without warning, the two of you are worlds apart. Utterly separate. Communication seems virtually impossible, and it almost feels as if you have stepped into a different personality. You hardly know yourself, let alone your lover. Moments before, he was here, right in front of you but now you are unable to meet his eyes, as though looking at him through a long tube. An overload of unexpressed feelings is activated, and you may suddenly feel in a fighting mood, blaming your partner for your unhappiness.

This is an immediate sign that emotions from the past have stepped in and temporarily disturbed your present moment. Although you may feel absolutely terrible, the truth is that facing such emotions can be beneficial because the experience is ultimately cleansing. I suggest that as soon as you recognize (and this gets easier and easier) what is happening, try to access the real feeling that the emotion is hiding or protecting. If you experience fear, you may find underneath that you feel utterly abandoned and alone; if you feel angry, you may find immense sadness. Allow the expression of this old buried feeling to overwhelm you.

If you cannot get back to it *immediately* acknowledge to yourself and your partner where you are, for instance: "I'm emotional right now, I'm feeling separate." But do not get engaged in any kind of blaming, or assume that *he* did the wrong thing. If talking about it improves the situation, it is helpful. But if the sense of separation persists, it is preferable to take some time alone.

What are you really feeling?

One distressing aspect of emotionality is that if one person gets emotional, it is not long before the second person is in a rage too, also accusing the other for countless disappointments! The situation has gone from bad to worse. The emotionality of one person will resonate and vibrate with the emotionality latent in the other, and so they inadvertently get involved in a conflict. Their repressed emotions are suddenly pouring out of every pore, and each one is blaming the other for it all! Communication can become absolutely impossible because neither person is clear or conscious. It is suggested that when you are very emotional, it is better not to talk because this rarely works out, and the confusion and separation often increase. Only if you are willing to *admit* to your vulnerability and *expose* it, should you carry on talking. Otherwise, it is far more respectful to acknowledge what is happening and to separate physically for a while. You can go for a walk and as little as an hour may be enough. Or you may need a longer time, a whole evening or a couple of days to give you time to work through the old emotions, expressing the feelings by having a good weep, or release feelings of rage and frustration by pounding a pillow. It is important to do something physical when you are emotional. Anything will do, such as jogging, dancing, or exercising.

Don't be afraid to give yourself adequate time, if you need it. During these moments of solitude, you may begin to notice that it is seldom this lover in particular who is entirely responsible for what you are experiencing, your sense of isolation, of being abandoned, rejected, betrayed. If you are honest with yourself, you will find you have had these feelings before. It's nothing new, only the scenario has changed, you even may notice it is a pattern which arises when you are growing in intimacy.

It is that excruciating experience of the heart wanting to open, but the hurt from another time, when you loved and were not loved in return, is there haunting you, keeping you withdrawn. We are all reliving the past in our present and this lover is not directly responsible for what you are going through. When you take full responsibility for your emotions, your love will not become contaminated with the unhappinesses of the past. When the right amount of time is taken for separation, the reunion can happen wordlessly as you step into the present.

It is by filtering these emotions from the genitals through the solar plexus to the heart, that they can be relived as real feelings and released. The emotion will sometimes be experienced on a physical level as a dense foreign substance swirling and spiraling uncomfortably within, flowing through the fascial system, which forms a weaving connective labyrinth throughout the body. Emotion clings to pride and protection and lacks the willingness to find the root of pain. If you have the courage to look beneath the emotion, however, your heart will race, your breath rate will increase, and you may shiver and sweat as you enter the reality of what you felt so long ago. Then your heart will speak of itself, its fragility and its tenderness. The wall between you and your lover will crumble right then and there. As suddenly as the emotion stepped in and separated you, it will leave. Your eyes can then meet those of your lover, and the sense of living in a separate reality will dissolve. Within these emotions is the kernel of our realignment with our essence, the love that we are.

Remember you are more than just your emotions

When you are in an emotional state, it is highly significant to realize that you are not your emotions, that you do not become over-identified with the pain and anguish of them, even though it can be hell. Do not trust anything that you do or say, either. Emotion likes revenge and you must avoid getting lost in there because this is not you. Do not do anything impulsive or potentially dangerous. Be aware of what you say. Understand what is happening, that a cloud of (past) emotion is overwhelming you. You need to be clear about the potential of men and women. As you let the sadness and pain emerge upward and out of the body try to cultivate an attitude of welcoming these feelings, understanding that you are unburdening your heart. This will bring a refreshing quality; you will feel more alive, closer to your lover and yourself

When we bring new intelligence to lovemaking, we come to understand the fluctuations from good to bad times. Learning to distinguish between emotions and feelings saves a lot of potential trouble when we can recognize repressed emotions creating a disturbance, sparking irritability, argumentativeness, and even physical excitement. It is crucial to understand that emotions create excitement. This is why sex is so hot and exciting while you are having a fight; the drama of it turns you on! Many couples will use sex as a last attempt to communicate, to patch up the pain of separation, but Tantra suggests that you never make love when you are in a fighting mood. It can easily lead to more emotion and therefore unconsciousness in sex. Wait until the emotions have passed before making love. Otherwise it is less easy to be aware as you make love, and difficult to meet in the loving and healing environment offered by the present. Since healing is a process, the fragile emotions can pop up unexpectedly at *any* moment, and if you are not alert, you're back in the ditch again, with the same story and the same issues.

Take every opportunity for greater expansion

When feelings arise, the mind can become a co-conspirator as it talks you out of sharing your feelings in order to avoid vulnerability. Once, ecstatically consumed by love, I wanted to say a simple, profound "I love you," but I could not bring myself to utter the words. I forcefully swallowed them. It was too intimate, too much in that moment or so my mind convinced me. It was not wise to reveal my love, vulnerability, or dependence. A few seconds later I felt my body begin to shrink, my presence collapsed, I was totally overcome with sadness. I wept, feeling my sexual energy and sensitivity slowly dwindle away. Shrunken and contracted I lay there flooded with all the accumulated memories of past moments when I had not expressed my love. In that excruciating pain of withholding, I saw how many opportunities I had missed that were doorways to greater expansion in body, heart, and spirit. Now, I use those precious gifts, and the heart soars on the wings of love.

On the journey from our personality to our being we will encounter layers of defense and protection and pain, which function to keep us away from our essence. These we have to meet and release as we take steps inward toward the core.

The following is a reliable guide to the different qualities of emotion and feeling, although some people admit to finding themselves in an ongoing low-grade emotional state, and these shifts are not detectable.

❀ *In emotion you will experience separation; in feeling you will experience closeness.*

❀ *Emotions are an unconscious expression; feelings are a conscious expression.*

❀ *Emotions usually refer to the past; feelings are experienced in the present.*

❀ *Emotion blames and projects: "you always/never...";* *feeling acknowledges: "I feel/need..."*

❀ *Emotion will repeat or use the same words year after year; feeling is expressed freshly.*

❀ *Emotion has exhausting effects; feelings expressed give vigor and life.*

❀ *Emotions represent the ego while feelings represent the heart.*

❀ *Emotions hang around for days; feelings expressed move on quickly.*

KEY POINTS:

❧ Feelings expand and connect us, while emotions contract and separate us.

❧ Emotions relate to our unexpressed past, feelings arise consciously in the present.

❧ Expressing feelings day by day prevents an emotional overload building up.

❧ Learning to identify "emotion" brings tremendous insight into relationship patterns. Remember, we are not our emotions.

❧ Old buried emotions are displaced through consciousness in lovemaking, welcome them.

23

WOMEN, EMOTIONS, AND THE HEART

WOMEN ARE WELL-KNOWN for their seemingly overwhelming emotions. The fact that emotions continually come to the surface even when everything seems to be going so well will often drive a man to despair. How can he love and understand a woman when harmony takes a sudden nosedive into depression, or flares up in a fight for no apparent reason? Women's irrational moods, arguing and nagging, questions and provocation, are a nightmare. It is as if the woman whom he loves so well is from time to time possessed.

The reasons for these emotional fluctuations lie in sex. Tantra teaches us that the emotional qualities that a man finds most disturbing in a woman are something that he himself actually creates through his insistence on excitement and orgasm. A woman is kept at the lowest level of her sexual expression and obstructed from fulfilling her true female potential. For centuries she has been used as a sexual object, the source of men's gratification. This saddens and enrages her. Over time her untapped divine energies become increasingly dormant and stagnant, while a deep dissatisfaction, disappointment, and lack of love pervades every cell in her body, making her emotionally unstable. Conventional sex, hot, frenzied, and focused on self-gratification, whips up these emotions within, and this triggers sexual excitement, interfering with her ability to be receptive.

Emotional sex and instability

Excitement deposits a residual tension in her body that affects both physical and psychological states, making her explosive and volatile with an instability, explaining why shortly after sex, couples can easily get into intense arguments. The sexual tension will be discharged sooner or later, like static electricity, and difficulties in relating will follow. Indeed, most relationship problems have their root in sexual dissatisfaction.

While emotional sex, as it is sometimes called, might be extremely pleasurable, it lasts only seconds, and ultimately has a depleting effect on the life energies. It can create dissatisfaction and a sense of separation where you no longer feel interested in your lover. Deep down we know we have used each other, not made love, and are saddened by it. This adds to our emotional store, rendering us unable to share love in the present as we live in the shadow of the past.

These emotional patterns and instability in a woman are so deeply ingrained that she begins to believe this is who she is. She has become identified with her emotional side. Women begin to falsely believe that a certain amount of emotion in their lives gives it shape, form, and meaning. They think that if there is a fight going on, then love is happening. Conversely and just as false, a woman often finds that if there is a period of calm and tranquillity between herself and her lover, then love must be disappearing. Often a woman will focus on an ongoing theme of discontent to get some attention and bring some life back into the relationship. She will create a bit of push and pull, a tug of war, just to get a sense of movement, a feeling of love.

When women are emotional, they become more excitable in sex, and this makes it difficult for both men and women to relax into making love. Orgasm will be a constant beckoning, pulling away from its spiritual nourishing phase. When the sexual energy is allowed to relax instead of being forced into a peak, the corresponding emotionality of a woman gradually subsides.

She is fulfilled, serene, and content. This is the shift from linear (sex energy released) to circular (sex energy retained) in which a woman finds herself more feminine, radiant, and loving. It is here in this circular movement, the union of sex and heart, where the true source of female sexual energy and ecstasy lies. Unfortunately women rarely reach their feminine potential because the crucial female polarity—awakening sex energy through the breasts and heart—in sex is not recognized or utilized either by herself or by her lover. Deep down she knows intuitively that much is possible from love and sex. She senses and longs for an orgasmic, blissful state of divine union where love reigns. But she remains fundamentally unsatisfied, and eventually her distress translates into emotionality.

As excitement and goal-oriented sex continue in her life, a woman will develop an emotional personality, demanding love and never finding the contentment of love within her. On the deepest level, this is a tragedy because we have lost our natural source of love. Excited, male-oriented sex never takes a woman to a state of true orgasmic bliss where her body pulsates with love energy and she feels herself as love itself. Furthermore, it begins to show up in the body, and sexual excitement forms a band of tension, which accumulates over the ovaries and uterus. Most women are not aware of this, but after years of heavy sex and forced orgasm, the ovaries and lower belly area become very congested and tense. This begins to disturb the health of a woman and she may find herself having repeated vaginal infections, irritations, or discharges, and it may even affect her urinary system. The breasts, which are not understood in terms of polarity, also begin to get diseased. Her hormones and menstrual cycle are affected too, thus her whole personality is influenced. The effects of these emotions are devastating and can leave a woman and her partner exhausted and confused for days. Love then becomes associated with the instability of constant ups and downs and a whirlwind of emotions.

Stepping away from emotional patterns

Tantra teaches us very clearly that love is not an emotion. Love is more a state of being, a quality that resides within you. It is cool not hot, accepting not challenging, relaxed not excited or tense, content not depressed. It is neither a demand nor an expectation, nor a contortion of the heart. Love illuminates, overflows, and radiates from within you. It is most valuable when a woman can begin to recognize when she is emotional, no matter how disappointed, angry, or jealous she may feel at that moment. Only then can she begin to step away from this intensity of overwhelming emotion, this disturbed aspect of her personality, and begin to create a new reality for herself where she is no longer victim but victor. She can tell her lover that she is feeling emotional and is not reliable or clear in that moment. Whatever she needs— a loving hug or some time alone—she can be vulnerable and ask for it. Her recognition of her emotionality can act as a constant reference point that she can use as a signal, to see the danger and turn the whole picture around before she gets caught up in it. This is taking real responsibility for love. Through taking conscious steps away from the emotion, and in so doing, cutting the unconscious patterns rooted in the past, a woman can begin to experience her deeper loving nature.

If a man is courageous enough to keep his sexual temperature to a cool burning flame and not a hungry fire, a woman will truly flower in her feminine sexual expression. When love is unhurried and allowed to manifest through polarity, men and women start to make love afresh. But this doesn't just happen; it requires vision, intelligence, and a commitment to love on the part of the man. Then he can help to reunite his lover with the divine source of her love in her body. When a man can see his woman blossom through his gathering of her divine energies, flower and radiate this love back to him, only then will he be truly satisfied with sex. Finally he feels within himself a true male authority. In the same way a woman can take responsibility for herself by insisting that a man make love to her, and not just have sex. In this clarity she prevents a further build up of debilitating emotions, and invites love back into her life. Unfortunately this can be difficult because women are so longing for love, that we will accept *any* attentions that masquerade in the name of love.

Making love in consciousness

It is good to be aware that when we are making love in consciousness, emotions will come and go in waves. Allow them to release through you, don't hold onto them. This is an intrinsic part of the internal balancing process. Women have more sexual wounds by virtue of their physical vulnerability, so it is natural they will face painful emotions more often. Even after a session of conscious lovemaking, it is common for women to be overcome with a wild irrational rage which they will be tempted to unleash on their lover, the same man they loved so much only an hour ago. Consciousness brought into the body must, and will, release these stored unconscious aspects within us. The silence instilled by consciousness in the body displaces these emotions. Allow these emotions to ride through your body freely, but do not direct them to or on your partner. Better to leave him out of it; take it back on yourself and enjoy the passion of it all. Go into a spare room and beat the hell out of a big cushion with your fists. Jump, dance, move! Be as physical as you can, but be aware of your body taking care not to hurt yourself accidentally.

During the healing which is initiated between penis and vagina, remember that a refining process is set in motion, as consciousness is instilled into the organs of love. Through a meditative approach in sex, a man can unite sex and heart in a woman, and reveal her essentially loving nature.

KEY POINTS:

෴ A man is largely responsible for the emotional fluctuations of a woman.

෴ Emotions have their source in the tensions of the conventional sex act.

217

ह∾Conscious sex reduces a woman's emotionality, her experience of separation between sex and love.

ह∾Acknowledging emotion is an essential step in restoring balance.

ह∾Through loving a woman a man can reveal a new world of love.

24

LIFE CYCLES AND
SAFE SEX

ALL OF NATURE IS BASED ON CYCLES of renewal
and retreat, waxing and waning, light and dark, birth
and death.

Sex cannot be separated from the dramatic event of birth,
while also being associated with a peaceful death. Birth implies
reproductive cycles and fertility cycles, both of which have a
profound influence on the life of a woman. Indeed, without
these cycles, we would not be here to celebrate the glory of love
and life. In the love arena, reproduction and fertility wreak
havoc. Just when things are wonderfully creative in love, there's
the interruption of menstruation or pregnancy.

Avoid unwanted pregnancy

It is essential that all women and men take adequate care not to
accidentally create another cycle of birth and death. It alters
lives. Today we are in the fortunate position of being able to
control birth in a variety of ways, and all people should
thoroughly inform themselves of the alternatives available by
seeking professional guidance. The insidious fear that a woman
carries buried within her—her capacity to be impregnated—
creates a deep and ongoing tension making it difficult for her to
relax fully into the sexual experience. Many women after being

sterilized have said this was their most striking liberation and made all the difference. It was an incredible relief even though most were not consciously aware of carrying this tension. A woman will also have the same experience if her lover has chosen to be sterilized himself by having a vasectomy.

When ejaculation frequency is reduced, this also reduces the chances of pregnancy. This is by *no* means saying that non-ejaculation is a substitute for contraception because seminal fluids are known to contain agile sperm. Nonetheless, one cannot help wondering if the population explosion today is a result of man's addiction to ejaculation. Condoms are often the simplest precaution that lovers can take. This applies in both new and long-term relationships.

Safe sex

When you make love with a new partner, condoms are also essential in the approach to safe sex—avoiding contracting sexually transmitted diseases including AIDS. To ensure protection genital body fluids must not be exchanged, so do not have *any* genital contact without a condom. You have to rely on yourself and it is imperative that you do not leave it up to somebody else. It is not worth the risk and discomfort that can follow. Always be prepared to speak to your partner about using a condom, whether you are a man or a woman. Keep some with you at all times. It is always beneficial to have an HIV test in order to allay any fears that you may have about AIDS. If a new friendship develops into a longer term partnership then both can be tested for HIV. The obvious answer for us today is to begin to make love to one person, and as we discover the true art of loving, we value the relaxation that comes with intimacy.

Condoms

However, condoms do represent an obstacle in the natural flow of events, when instead of penetration there is encapsulation, and the whole affair can shrink into folds of dismal shriveled rubber. This does mean that couples and lovers need to talk about it in advance to avoid unfortunate situations. Particularly if experimenting within new guidelines, such communication is essential. It is always a relief when sex is out in the open and fears dissolve, creating relaxation and rapport.

So tell your partner what your circumstances are and what works for you. Ask for any help you need, offer any assistance they might need. If it is not appropriate for you to make love, it might be better to wait till another time. It can happen that you lose your erection whilst applying a condom, but do not lose heart. After a few minutes start afresh and apply the condom to the unerect penis. If you continue with foreplay and awakening to each other sexually, your penis is likely to rise in response, and you can continue.

Generally speaking it is better to place the condom on at the outset of making love, well before you have an erection. It is possible to place a condom on a soft or semi-soft penis, and this can be done by the man or the woman, or both! Roll the foreskin back and pull all the folds of skin toward the base of the penis, so as to reveal the head. Roll on the condom, slowly, pulling it all the way down. From here, your penis can gradually become erect within the condom, and when the right moment for penetration presents itself, you can proceed accordingly!

People often ask if the rubber of a condom inhibits sensitivity. Yes, undoubtedly it does, as there is an undeniable layer between the penis and its delicate environment. However, the intrinsic sensitivity of the penis remains unaffected as men report the same miraculous magnetic response of the penis within the vagina regardless of this lack of true physical contact. This is undeniable proof of the finesse and intelligence of the penis.

Lubricants

Condoms are *only* to be used with special pharmaceutical lubricant such as KY Jelly, or "designer-style" lubricants that have an aqueous base (water). Condoms must not be used with vegetable oil or petroleum jelly, which destroy the rubber and compromise protection. (Condoms are also known to tear or disintegrate for no apparent reason.) There are many lubricants on the market; find one that suits you. Oil was used by the Chinese Taoists centuries ago and it was said to keep down the level of bacteria. A pure unscented vegetable or nut oil (such as almond oil) is fine but remember, not in conjunction with condoms. Saliva is good for emergencies, it has the most wonderful texture of all, but it is not always clean. Introducing saliva into the vagina can therefore upset the natural acid-alkali balance and irritations can occur.

Be sensitive during menstruation

The onset of menstruation triggers different responses in men and women. There are no general rules. Each couple has to be sensitive to the needs of the other, and decide according to their situation. Women often have heightened sensitivity at this time and may dread being deserted, while men fear the blood or the mess of it all. Be loving with each other nonetheless, share and exchange energy in bodily embraces or lie silently and rest in consciousness together. Such moments can be penetrating too.

While menstruating, it is recommended that the woman assume a position on top of the man to support the menstrual flow by not reversing it, which can have congesting effects. Heavy thrusting is not recommended at this time either. A conventional orgasm is known to dispel the tensions of menstrual pain, but this is only a short-term measure as the pain is often a reflection of gathered sexual tensions. So, make it a gentle relaxed orgasm so that you do not reinforce the tensions already present. As a woman begins to relax in lovemaking, she is likely to find a corresponding improvement in problems with menstrual pain, and indeed in her all her premenstrual and menstrual syndromes. Her general outlook on life will be enhanced and she will also feel herself giving and receiving love more easily.

As we make love we may notice that interest or intensity in lovemaking comes and goes. There seem to be cycles of extreme intensity suddenly followed by a plateau. These are the rhythms of nature, where rest always follows activity, and should not cause doubt or resentment. However, even when we do not apparently feel like making love, it is recommended to try it out. Put the bodies together and see what happens. Often the mind is not prepared to be present and relaxed, while in contrast the body is usually more than willing. Remember you can stop at any time. So many surprising experiences happened when I apparently did not feel like making love. So it can often be more beneficial to make love than to make an excuse.

A woman often feels distressed and emotional in the days before the onset of menstruation. In fact life can be hell for her and she is filled with doubt and insecurity. In this state she usually considers lovemaking an impossibility because at heart she feels unlovable. If a man can encourage her to make love consciously, many of her tensions and insecurities will disperse through the sexual exchange. Calmness and contentment will prevail and menstruation will become less of a torment. It is very important that a man be direct with a woman when she has an emotional crisis during her premenstrual or menstrual period. The man must avoid getting emotional too, by way of unconscious reaction, but remind the woman lovingly what is happening to her, and offer his support. For instance "What do you need right now?"

"What I can I do for you?" Physical contact is ever-healing because deep down the woman is missing love—the reason underlying all emotionality.

Make love if you can, because love is the greatest therapy there is, it works miracles. Support her through the crisis, be with her and be loving, do not abandon or blame her. A man has much to answer for in his addiction to sexual excitement. It has eroded away the essential qualities of a woman and she can so easily be unstable and unpredictable in turn. His task today is to reverse this process. With a new vision, old wounds can be healed through communication and consciousness, and men and women are encouraged to be as open as possible and say how they feel.

While the hormonal cycles of women are well known and well discussed, the lesser-known hormonal cycles of men lie unacknowledged. Evidence gradually emerges to indicate that there are subtle cycles that affect men at a deeper level, and men do get the blues! It is no wonder with love being in such disarray. It is his partner's hormonal cycles that have the most subterranean impact on him, and in his ignorance, he reinforces this. When she is tied up in hormonal knots, and as a man he is unable to reach her, this affects his mind and body profoundly. On the other hand, when he becomes more aware in sex, his partner will respond by being more loving; she will be sexually more available to him. This expression of his masculinity has a strengthening influence, and without habitual ejaculation the hormonal factors stimulated by sexual activity will be reabsorbed, translating into physical vitality and a loving heart. Sex is an uplifting, energizing force.

Cycles of ill-health

While it may seem a little unrelated, it is important to mention cycles of genital ill-health. Many couples that have experimented with reducing excitement and tension in sex have found a corresponding reduction in repetitious genital infections. Both men and women can suffer from ongoing genital disturbances including candida, herpes, cystitis, bladder infections, thrush, and mysterious discharges or irritations. Couples have noticed a distinct change in the pattern of such occurrences once consciousness is introduced into lovemaking. It seems that as the genital tissues become polarized, relaxed, and healthier, irritations of the sexual organs diminish. A friend, who had been plagued by such occurrences for several years, said to me "My vagina is now totally healthy. Before that it was a constant struggle against herpes and candida. It is really amazing. I feel so happy about this because it was really a burden for me, for our sexual life and the relationship."

Similarly, a close male friend suffered from herpes. It followed him like a shadow, a constant source of distress, and he felt his manhood threatened by his lack of availability. Once he began to make love with more awareness and a more loving, respectful attitude to himself and his woman, he observed that his outbreaks of herpes diminished. He began to notice that if he let go into his conditioning, making love without consciousness, that a herpes outbreak would follow almost immediately. As the process of staying present and conscious deepened for him, the recurring outbreaks stopped. When it happened unexpectedly, he was always able to trace it back to some unexpressed emotion, something he did not allow himself to feel.

Bladder infections in women can often be the result of vigorous sex. The friction irritates the urethral opening just below the clitoris, and so a site for infection is created. Bladder infections will frequently occur when a couple have been separated for a while and upon reunion they make love with a great deal of energetic enthusiasm rather than renewed, relaxed sensitivity. Friction produces a tension in men and women, which eventually disturbs the genital tissues. The charge has no way of flowing out of the energy system so it builds up and manifests as physical irritations or disturbances.

Relaxation is the ever-healing force. As the finesse of lovemaking increases and the sexual tensions relax, a rearrangement of sexual energy takes place, enabling it to flow along inner ecstatic pathways. This has a profound impact on the psyche, and harmony of body and spirit follows. We are able to transcend the biological life cycle of reproduction and expand into the spiritual generative cycle of the sexual energy, fulfilling our human potential. This is the greatest life cycle of all, where sex is used to instill awareness of life beyond the body, and beyond life itself.

KEY POINTS:

ॐ Sexual energy and interest is subject to natural cycles.

ॐ Explore making love even when you don't "feel like it".

ॐ Contraception and safe sex must be talked about in advance.

ॐ Non-ejaculation is not a substitute for contraception or safe sex.

ॐ Loving sensitivity and communication is required during menstruation.

25

ALONE OR
ON YOUR OWN

WHEN WE FIND OURSELVES ALONE or without a
lover, we may well ask: What do I do with my sexual
energy now? How do I stay vibrant and sensuous?
How can I invite love into my life? Tantra reminds us that each
man or woman is a complete unit within themselves. Recalling
the theme of polarity, a man's body carries a positive pole in
the penis and a negative pole in the heart, while a woman's body
is negative in the vagina and positive in the breasts and heart.
These opposite poles form a rod of magnetism, which means
that energy can be circulated between this positive and negative,
and this circulation happens independently. The joy and ecstasy
felt during deep orgasm happens within your very own body
and is dependent on your own inner sensitivity and awareness.
This explains, for instance, why a woman may report having
an orgasmic experience while her partner was half-asleep and
uninvolved. The simple fact of the penis lying *in* the vagina
triggers the internal energy movement. If the person is very alive
to themselves, this is enough to bring them into a blissful state.

If we have had one single orgasmic experience in sex where
the sexual energy moves orgasmically inward and upward,
Tantra tells us that this very experience can be used to increase
consciousness. By recreating this internally, by consciously

moving the awareness within the body, a vibrating cellular experience can be recalled and relived again and again. Through this conscious reliving of the orgasmic state, the orgasmic energy flowing within, great transformation is possible. So it is wonderful to realize that you can consciously prolong the beneficial effects of lovemaking through the power of imagination.

If you are separated from your lover for a while, you can set aside a specific time to lie down and attune to yourself and your inner electricity. Use the imagination to support the energy flow through the body. Very soon you will start to feel a streaming through the body not unlike when you are making love. It will have a similar quality. It is also good to use this as a way of communicating with your lover instead of relying on the telephone as we often do and finding words hopelessly inadequate. Instead, make an agreement or date to lie down and relax at exactly the same time, say, nine o'clock at night. You are separated physically but are together in spirit. Fifteen to twenty minutes is enough, but you can try longer too. You will be amazed at the loving and refreshing results. Through this practice you are reinforcing the love to be found within yourself, the love that is an expression of your being.

Resting in consciousness

If you are alone and without a partner, this circulation of vital energy within your body is possible. It is highly recommended because it turns the awareness inward to bring yourself into focus. This in itself is a tremendous nourishment and you will find yourself feeling more loving and content. To have Tantra in your life while you are alone, all it takes is to make some undisturbed time each day to lie down and rest. The idea is to *rest* and take the consciousness into the body. When we achieve this union with the subtle energies in the body, time melts away and inner contentment arises. We feel filled up, and not the empty space in bed next to us. However, this requires that we remain conscious.

Most of us, when we go to sleep at night or have a nap, use

it as time to escape the pressures of reality, and check out for a while. Often after this kind of rest, you awaken feeling a bit drugged, and the worse for it— it did not give you the refreshment you were seeking. We all know too, how it feels to wake up in the morning and feel quite exhausted, as though we haven't slept. Bringing consciousness to the body can eliminate these effects.

Resting in consciousness *(see* fig. 16) is perhaps the most delightful and beneficial thing people can do for themselves on a regular, even daily, basis. It needs a minimum of twenty minutes. It is as simple as this: lie down, close your eyes, and bring the consciousness to reside within your body. Lie with the spine, head, and neck in straight line. This alignment is crucial because it contributes tremendously to your presence. Place a supporting pillow under the knees so that they are slightly softened and bent. This really enhances relaxation, and enables your consciousness to move beyond the physical boundaries of the body.

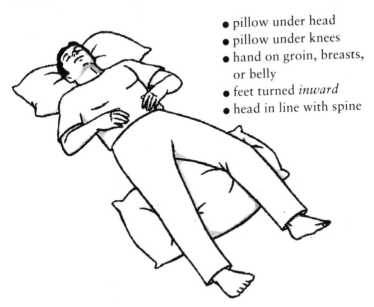

- pillow under head
- pillow under knees
- hand on groin, breasts, or belly
- feet turned *inward*
- head in line with spine

Fig. 16   Resting in consciousness

Once you are comfortable, turn your attention from outside to inside, leaving behind the thoughts of the day. Sweep through your whole body with your awareness, softening and relaxing any tensions you may feel. It can help to contract and tighten the body at first, exaggerating the tensions. Do this several times, tighten and release. Sense the upper half of the body and then the lower half of the body, and unite them with your consciousness in the area above the navel. Slowly sink into the sensations of the body, looking inward and down with your inner eye at the same time. Spread it evenly throughout the entire body. Keep the head and neck in line. Breathe deeply and slowly and "be." Do this for twenty minutes only. At a certain moment you may slip into yourself, into timelessness. Observe how incredibly rejuvenated you feel after such a rest! It is quite miraculous. If you do this before you sleep at night, and take the first twenty minutes to rest in consciousness, you will find the quality of your sleep to be more refreshing. Indeed, you may even require less sleep. Resting itself can become a rejuvenating meditation when you are horizontal, a most delightful position. Turning inward gets easier with practice, and resting in consciousness becomes an incredible life support, as its effects are most beneficial. When relaxation arises through consciousness it becomes a healing and energizing force.

How to connect with your inner opposite pole

To deepen this meditation and take it further, slowly bring your positive pole into awareness and imagine golden light filling the area. Women should focus on both nipples simultaneously, and men should focus on the perineum at the root of the penis. Once you have a feeling of light or energy building up, you can begin to imagine this light overflowing, spreading and streaming toward the opposite negative pole. Women may experience this as a gradual spreading and rising of energy, while men may feel it as leaps or jumps of light or energy moving upward. Connecting in this way with our inner opposite pole, our own magnetic rod, an increasingly ecstatic circle of energy is formed within. It may take time to build up to this, and if you have been fortunate enough to have had one previous ecstatic sexual experience where the energy turned orgasmically inward, use your awareness to provoke this memory in the cells of your body. You can add the breath to this meditation on the positive poles: a woman can imagine herself breathing in through the vagina and out through the heart, and a man can imagine breathing in through the heart and out through the penis.

Women in particular should meditate on the positive pole, the breasts and nipples. This activates the feminine energies inherent in the breasts and begins to rebalance the polarity. As the breasts themselves begin to get energized, the heart center begins to vibrate and expand, enveloping her with great sweetness. It is recommended however, that a woman brings her awareness into the nipples (both simultaneously), and not to the heart center itself. The idea is to open the heart *through* the breasts, which has a profound impact on a woman's energy system and spreads through the whole body. When a woman is alone and finds herself sorely missing love, meditating on the breasts can become a powerful support. This keeps the feminine energy awakened and vital, and the inward turning of the awareness positively diverts the energy she might otherwise pour into longing for love. As life would have it, in so doing she begins to shine and becomes attractive. Many women have had the experience that love came to them the very moment they stopped searching for it, when they finally gave up. As soon as they accepted the situation and felt loving toward themselves, love would knock on the door and walk right in and stay.

This gives a clue to us all, men and women, that self-love is crucial. We cannot ask another to love us without loving ourselves first, without being willing to give love, which also means having enough love within ourselves to share. When you bring consciousness into the body, a feeling of lovingness and tenderness toward oneself is generated; one is more present and graceful. Anything that you enjoy in the way of exercise, massage, bodywork, or dancing is very healthy when done regularly and is tremendously supportive in enhancing body sensitivity and awareness.

Be receptive to the growing consciousness in your body

To support the growing of consciousness in the body, use the Love Keys. Many of them can be used outside of sex with good effect, like slowing down when we eat, relaxing as we clean our teeth, walking slowly. When we find ourselves alone, it is very useful to remember to relax the pelvic floor, breathe, allow the vision to be inward and outward at the same time. By using the awareness, many of the Love Keys can be incorporated into your life, and this relaxation will bring a qualitative change to your daily routine. You may find you achieve more with less effort. While washing the dishes for instance, try standing equally weighted on both feet with the knees slightly bent. This immediately creates a physical presence and grounding, the warm watery soapy suds are unexpectedly a sensual joy. The chore can suddenly seem effortless as the body aligns itself with the force of gravity.

When we stand with all our body weight on one leg, knee joint locked and out of alignment, we feel unwilling and heavy while time seems to drag. In the same way, when chatting at a cocktail party, waiting in line at the airport, theater, or bank, practice again and again standing on both feet equally, letting the knees be soft and the body weight relax down into the pelvis, legs, and feet. You may notice that you suddenly feel more attentive, present, and receptive. Your impatience and dissatisfaction will dissolve as you begin to respond to the small amusing and colorful details present in almost every scene. Be present to your environment, absorb your surroundings, notice everything around you but without losing awareness of yourself. It is as if you perceive the outside through the inside. This heightens your sensitivity as you are seated within yourself as if at home.

As we bring the internal circulation of our vital energy into practice, there will be a possible corresponding rise in sexual energy, or life energy. Enjoy the sensation of this aliveness in your body. Do not be afraid to feel sexual, this is the juice of life, and do not think you have to do something with this energy to release it. Contain it and concentrate it within you, and wait for love to arrive in your life. Do not seek it or expect it, but invite it. Look again, and you will find love in the smallest of things.

It may happen that the need or urge arises for self-pleasuring, or masturbation, and this is because our sexual energy is continually seeking expression. The urge can also represent a certain level of sexual tension or excitement present in the system. Nonetheless, it is important to remember that masturbation is fertile soil for fantasy, has little to do with the real thing, and can be a hindrance to consciousness. In lovemaking the focus is on relaxation and this should also be the focus of self-pleasuring. Use the Love Keys to guide you. As you touch and caress yourself, avoid building up any sexual tension or urgency. Instead, stroke yourself unhurriedly including your buttocks, legs, and feet. Slowly reabsorb each lingering touch. Touch and be aware of the touch at the same time—this will intensify your presence and experience. Breathe deeply and continuously, spread the energy around the body, roll about and celebrate your sensuality. If the need for an orgasm persists, then prolong the self-touching. Don't be in a hurry to reach the end. When you do orgasm or ejaculate, be aware of what is happening as it is happening and relax into the experience of it. If you can, place one hand on your heart. Avoid using sexual images but if necessary it is suggested the man imagine the vagina only, or the woman, the penis. This keeps the emphasis on where love is actually made between penis and vagina, rather than vivid sexual imagination, which is exciting and provocative.

Men have reported that, much to their surprise, after a time of making love in a conscious way the interest in masturbation diminished. After the penis had been experienced as a generator of energy, and sexual energy as a glowing force, it became of no intrinsic value.

Begin a new relationship in consciousness

If you meet someone and you wish to make love, explain that you are interested in trying something different. It may seem a bit of a daunting prospect but it is good not to delay it. If you are able to begin your sex life with an element of consciousness, it has a far greater chance of strengthening into love. It is very important too that women begin to choose consciousness and stop compromising with men, because they do so at their own expense. The mind will nonetheless try and convince you to do it in the usual way for a while and postpone talking about it until later. However, the emotional reactions spawned by unconscious sex are often so fast, unpredictable, and overwhelming that frequently we are separated before we know it! Love does not have a chance to take root let alone get off the ground, because sexual energy is misunderstood and this has consequences.

Don't be afraid to introduce the subject of sex, because deep down everybody is vulnerable. We are all confounded by it. Usually it is a relief, a relaxation to talk of our feelings and get sex out in the open. Share what you understand so far and make suggestions as to how to proceed in a new way. Talk about the Love Keys and see which you can immediately begin to use. Start with a slow approach and take your time, avoiding excitement or focus on orgasm. I have found the response to relaxation astounding.

A friend of mine who enjoyed changing partners at one time explained to a new woman how he wanted to make love with her; very slowly, with eye contact, and without excitement or orgasm. The results were amazing! Each time, the woman experienced a tremendous opening in her body and heart, falling in love with him immediately. The love generated by a conscious penis is instantaneous and a woman is exceptionally sensitive to its tremendous power. So rarely does she experience it in consciousness, that when she does, she knows and wants more of it! She feels encountered and fulfilled for the first time, and the first penetration can be enough. In the same way, once a man tastes his sexual energy as a divine moving force, nothing else truly satisfies him.

Sometimes in a couple, partners will get the urge to be on their own for a while or "have some space" because the exchange with the other is experienced as a demand or as needy or tiring. When the focus of the lovemaking is turned inward and away from habitual orgasm, couples report that this imbalance shifts and there arises a contentment with silence and quiet moments between them, with each one more centered and at home, as if alone together.

KEY POINTS:

ટ≫ Vital energy can be circulated in the body while alone.

ટ≫ Resting in consciousness is profoundly relaxing and rewarding.

ટ≫ Energize the positive poles with the awareness.

ટ≫ Most Love Keys can be used in daily life to great effect.

ટ≫ When you meet someone new, start experimenting right away.

26

THE LOVE
TEMPLE

THE AMBIENCE OF A ROOM, its scent and flavor, can remind you of the sacredness of lovemaking. It can have an air about it that evokes love and instills reverence. It can remind you that you are here in love, for love, and to love. If you design your bedroom around lovemaking with the bed as the focal point, you will soon begin to feel a wave of awe and sensuality pass through you upon entering. If you have a date to make love, then purify and clean the room some hours before, giving it your loving touch. Then it will be like a temple, the perfect atmosphere for the celebration of love.

If you have the luxury of a spare room, turn it into your love temple, keeping it for these special occasions. Remove as much of the furniture as possible, and pictures, photographs, and knick-knacks from the past. The idea is to create a tranquil spaciousness that will assist and invite you into the clarity of the present moment. If you have no extra room, remove all the unnecessary stuff from your bedroom. Create the feeling of an empty space. Ornaments and family photographs gather dust and become invisible after a while, giving a room an overfilled, stuffy, or chaotic feeling. Fewer things in your room will make it feel bigger, providing you with a sense of expansion. An Italian couple that had been married for twenty-five years took my course. When they arrived home again, they found they simply *had* to change the furniture layout in their house so that a fresh environment could support their new commitment to love. By removing the redundant clutter of family memorabilia, they regained the ability to see each other anew.

Create a special atmosphere to make love

Lighting makes all the difference to a room; it's great to have lots of options. Try using four or five different lights, different colors creating a soft, warm effect while at the same time making sure you have enough light to be able to see into the eyes of your partner. Although sometimes it is glorious to make love in the intimacy of darkness, initially it is easier to stay present when you can see each other well. The flickering flame of candlelight always brings a special quality to the atmosphere even if there are other lights on at the same time. If you use only candles, which is also very nice, use many so as to fill the room with dancing flames.

Soft music creates a soothing ambience and warms the heart before and as you make love. This is where auto-reverse tape and CD players really come in handy; put on something you both like and let it go around until the lovemaking is over. At the same time, making love in silence has its merits. I have found that music can also act as a screen, a place to get lost. So although it may feel awkward at first with no sounds to support and inspire you, it is good to make love in silence as well, so the awareness is literally forced into the body.

It is great to have a big bed or a huge mattress on the floor, the bigger the better, so you are not afraid to roll around and be playful. Low, large beds are perfect for split-level positions giving one the distinctly feline feeling of lounging stretched out, half on, half off the bed. Plenty of bed space allows you to move around together in rotation positions that enhance the genital communion and depth of penetration. A firm mattress is a good idea, providing solid ground for your bodies. If the mattress is very soft and collapses in the middle, it will be difficult to find and maintain different positions.

You both need to be well supported and comfortable, so let your bed be a constant invitation, which you can't resist. Bed linens of gorgeous design, color, and quality can make slipping into bed a glorious and sensuous experience. And have plenty of pillows too, so they can be used later to support different parts of the body while you're making love. For example, when a woman is lying on her back, she can place a pillow beneath her hips to raise the level of her pelvis allowing for deeper penetration. If you are making love sitting up, the woman in the lap of her partner with her legs around his pelvis (the Yab Yum position), a pillow under her buttocks can make it more comfortable and the genital contact more penetrating. In the same way, legs, knees, heads, and necks sometimes need extra support.

Plants and flowers add a touch of color and beauty to the environment. If you are planning a special night together, perhaps an anniversary or other celebration, fill the room with heaps of colorful flowers, especially roses, which touch the heart. The fragrance helps you to remain in your senses, while it may also remind you to breathe more easily and fully. Fragrance can be felt as the room wrapping itself around the body, so incense and aromatic lamps or candles can bring a special quality. I always feel that I am being embraced by the atmosphere when the air is filled with incense. After a few occasions, a particular scent will become associated with love, and as you step into the room you will feel an opening within, a wonderful readiness for love.

I've always liked mirrors in a room to reflect and amplify the surroundings. There is nothing wrong with enjoying the reflection of you and your lover's bodies relaxing together, indeed it is beautiful, but be aware that mirrors can stimulate your sexual imagination. Mirrors can be better used to bring the outside in. By placing a mirror opposite a window with a view, you get the view twice or even more. I once managed to use the placement of mirrors to reflect the illusion of eighty-eight flames from only eleven candles. Rather than using one complete mirror that is heavy and hard to handle, use strips of mirror, anything from two inches to six inches wide, with a pencil-thick gap between them. This has the glorious effect of breaking up the reflection, amplifying it and opening up a whole new visual world within your bedroom. Do whatever appeals to you, whatever feels magical and sensual, so that when you step into your room the flickering candles and soft music will remind you of a temple: serene, quiet, fragrant, and flower-filled.

As you prepare your environment, prepare the body to make love in consciousness, which requires a step down into the senses. Leave the activities and concerns of the day behind. A warm shower or a relaxing hot bath is really the best thing one can do before making love, finishing off with a splash of refreshing cold water if you are brave. Water is just marvelous because it washes away stale, congested energy, and you emerge refreshed with your energy cleansed and more present in body and spirit. Some movement is helpful, as is breathing or quiet meditation, all of which help bring consciousness to the body.

A beautiful way to start and finish making love is with a *namaste*. This is the classic hand-gesture of India, with the palms together in a prayer position and held in front of the heart. It is accompanied by a slight bowing of the head. Traditionally the meaning of this gesture is "I greet the Buddha in you." It is also known as the heart *mudra*, and activates the heart center. Before you begin to make love, sit opposite each other, eyes meeting, and take a bow. Acknowledge yourself and each other, and bow your heads in acknowledgment of the blessings flowing from presence. It creates an awareness of what you are entering into. Often after extraordinary sexual union, you will find yourself spontaneously bringing your hands together in this heart *mudra* in sheer gratitude to your lover for the heartfelt experience. It is almost an instinctive response. Gracefully complete the lovemaking with a bow as you feel the joy and peace that arises when love has truly been made, a peace that passes all understanding.

Some people like ritual to help them create a new and different atmosphere for making love. Ritual is like opening a doorway leading to specific steps that encourage you into the experience of the present moment, through the body and the senses. It does not work for everyone, but for some, rituals or practices can be very powerful in establishing an energetic field to support their presence, so you might like to create your own personal way of preparing for love. As you perform this sequence again and again, the effect of the ritual or practice will soon resonate in your body and prepare you for an inner journey.

Finally, let your precious presence bring grace to your environment wherever you are. Let your body serve as a constant reminder of the consciousness that can be brought to love and sex. The body is the finest and most graceful temple on earth, and to find God within oneself, through sex, is the great gift of life.

KEY POINTS:

ॐ Beauty and fragrant surroundings invoke the senses and inspire you.

ॐ Design yourself a dream bed so it is a constant invitation to love.

ॐ Use lighting, music, flowers, and fragrance to create ambience.

ॐ The body is the greatest temple when radiant with presence.

The following meditation can be used as a preparation for lovemaking or to bring lovers closer when there is a feeling of separation.

CIRCLE OF LIGHT BREATHING— MEDITATION ON LIGHT

Meditation on light is one of the most ancient Tantric meditations. The moment you meditate on light, something inside you that has remained a bud starts opening its petals. The meditation on light creates a space for its opening.

Prepare your room as a temple with flowers, music, and incense.

Place candles around the room, creating enough light to see the eyes of your lover.

In the center of the room place a mattress on the floor with a pillow at each end of the mattress so that it is possible to sit opposite each other.

Between the two pillows place one candle.

Be sure there is enough space between the pillows so that you can sit comfortably and have the candle between you.

Choose a piece of music (about forty-five minutes long) that opens and expands your energy.

Place additional cushions or chairs at opposite ends of the room, well away from the central area.

Prepare the room in advance and leave it empty for half an hour with music playing during this time.

Take a shower and then meet your lover in silence at the door of the temple wearing comfortable, loose clothing, which you can later remove if you wish.

Start the chosen tape or CD, or leave it playing as you find it upon entering.

Walk slowly to the two cushions or chairs placed at opposite ends of the room, and sit in meditation for about ten to fifteen minutes.

Close your eyes and allow a quality of stillness to arise within. Forget about your lover and bring the attention to yourself.

Slide your awareness down your spine and into your belly.

Breathe in to a point two inches below your navel.

Breathe out to the count of three.

Breathe in to the count of three.

Keep your awareness in your belly.

Breathe for several minutes in this way.

When you have the feeling of yourself "arriving" in your body, allow your eyes to open.

Let the vision be soft and inward, as if the temple is looking into you. Slowly come to a standing position, feeling your legs and feet as roots to the ground.

Bring intense awareness to the penis (man) and breasts (woman) so as to awaken the energy within.

Slowly start to walk toward the place of worship.

The slower you walk the better, experiencing yourself more as energy than body.

Sit down opposite each other on the mattress, looking at the candle flame between you.

As you breathe in, imagine you are breathing in the light.

The woman is breathing in through the vagina and out through the heart.

The man is breathing out through the penis and in through the heart.

Allow the light to circulate through your own body breathing in synchronicity, as if the breath is speaking to your lover.

When you feel that you are filled with light, raise your eyes to meet your lover and exchange energy through the eyes.

After some moments, the man removes the

candle between you, the woman moves across
the space to sit in the Yab Yum position.

Continue to breathe in synchronicity, the
woman in through the vagina and out through
the heart, the man in through the heart and out
through the penis, circulating the light.

Continue to breathe and circulate light until the
music finishes. In due course, slowly separate
and worship your lover, giving thanks
and gratitude with a *namaste* (bow).

Lie down together and relax, or make love.

*Sex is one of the activities given by nature and God in which
you are thrown again and again to the present moment.
Ordinarily you are never in the present—except when you are
making love, and then too for a few seconds only. Tantra says
one has to understand sex, to decode sex. If sex is so vital that
life comes out of it, then there must be something more to it.
That something more is the key towards Divinity, towards God.*
Osho, The Tantra Vision

AFTERWORD

WHEN I FIRST HAD THE URGE to write a book, I promised myself that it would be short. What I felt at the outset and increasingly since, is that the essentials of sex are simple and elementary, even while vastly complex in implication. Most of what I had seen on sex did not seem simple at all. To find more it appeared that I would have to compound effort with effort. The truth I discovered was that in doing less I found more. Sex is astonishingly simple because the male and female human bodies are beautifully and ingeniously crafted to connect, one slipping into the other with the power to generate a divine biological ecstasy, lifting us into the dimension of love and meditation very naturally, an essential for regeneration of the spirit. We need sex in the same way we need air and water. In the absence of this vital energy flowing within, we feel as a hollow shell, dragging the stiffened body, weary in spirit, desolate at heart. Sex is our link with the divine, our key to the alchemy of energy and the mysteries of life.

Our privilege in being human is to generate this ecstatic energy in consciousness, and it is this consciousness that distinguishes us from the animal kingdom. Even though we have much to learn from the observation of animal love-play, they do lack a "consciousness" of themselves, ecstatically present to the splendor of the moment only in instinct. Perhaps this has influenced us in dismissing sex as a purely instinctive animal function, devoid of spirit. And yet we embody both, with our animal aspect fulfilled through procreation, the descending half of the circle of sexual energy, and through inverting this *same* energy, the ascending spiritual phase arises where an ecstatic sexual energy is generated.

The widespread conditioning has belittled sex and we have been denied the ecstatic spiritual part of it. Sex is viewed superficially as a physical or emotional need, and so we feign disinterest in it while our hearts are confused, making us afraid to bring it out in the open. We ignore sex, while other obsessions and compulsions arise in compensation. Yet we are still driven by the unconscious forces of sex. From time to time we have "to do it" and then we keep it hidden and in the dark. An immediate purpose is served, congestion is dispersed, but it fails to be a genuine sexual experience of love.

Several men have told me that when they were young and first sexual, their impulse was to lie effortlessly inside the vagina. That is what they really wanted to do. And then later, most dismayed, they saw the movies, heard the gossip, looked at magazines, and forced themselves to make a concerted effort in sex, painfully turning away from their blissful nature. It has been my observation that the younger a person is, the more easily they are able to step aside from or deflect the influences of our sexual conditioning, to connect with their innocence. However, as the years pass by, the shell of conditioning cast around us toughens, fears grow, tensions solidify in a physical form, resignation steps in, we become attached to our ways and so complacency keeps us held in many unconscious patterns. But the beauty is that this sexual misunderstanding can be dissolved with consciousness; that is all that is needed, and it works. And the sooner we can start, the better. There are very few resilient individuals who are what can be called "naturally Tantric" and fortunate enough to retain this God-given sexual innocence throughout their existence, while some will require only one profound Tantric experience to completely transform their lives. For others, to find their way back to this sexual simplicity can be described as a slow erosion, a gradual shift from dark to light, delightfully traveling all the shapes and contours in between.

Only *through* making love was I able unravel the misunderstandings *about* making love. It was not talking about it or thinking about it that made the difference, it was actually *doing* it that made the difference. Talking about how you wish to make love, and then holding to it *while* making love, are vastly different. As soon as the bodies are united, these unconscious patterns begin their play and we can find the ideals we started out with may not be so easy to stay with. The unconscious forces in the body are so much stronger than our presence and consciousness in the beginning, and they are persistent. We are where we are. It is a process of bringing the sexual experience slowly and surely into consciousness, learning to relate out of the sexual here and now. The urge to "go for coming" would arise for me soon after, if not before I was penetrated. My body and psyche was so accustomed to responding to the urge, that it took me time to adjust my mind and unhook the bodily reactions that pulled me down the track automatically. As my interest in orgasm was released, slowly my body was able to respond naturally out of each moment, to find that each time was unique.

To bring these shifts of consciousness into play to qualitatively change your love experience requires that you make love with the same person again and again. It is a gradual attunement of two divine instruments, slowly bringing them into fine harmony with each other. As time passes, finesse grows; the magnetic poles align and melt ecstatically into each other.

It certainly requires commitment on the part of a couple, and doesn't happen by accident unless you are lucky. It is as if a switch has to be turned on, which is the simplest thing in the world, but we have forgotten the knack, so we need practice. First and foremost, the commitment must be to now, this time and not the next. When I first started experimenting it began as a day-to-day affair so I never had a choice but *now,* this very time to make love. It forced me into the present, there was a sense of urgency, no opportunity to be lost, and I can say that this strengthened my consciousness. I had to make love as beautifully and as consciously as possible *now,* and not tomorrow. Tomorrow never comes. Willingness, flexibility, a preparedness to play around, and a humorous side are required to start all over again. Be willing to experience yourself in a refreshing new way. To enable this to unfold within, to teach yourselves as a couple, means having courage to experiment and to share experiences during lovemaking, and to talk about it afterward as well. Perhaps even in descriptive detail. Any level of intimacy reached with your lover will be reflected as increased sensitivity and pleasure while lovemaking.

Remember to observe what happens to you after lovemaking; how you feel in your body, your emotional state, how close you feel to your lover. The answers to these inner questions will begin to give you clues and guidelines about the essential spirit of lovemaking, and how to maintain love and harmony in your life. It may seem for the first time you have a glimpse of what it means to love. True learning comes out of experience. One time you may feel "blissed out", the next bitchy and unhappy. Why? What happened during the lovemaking that made you feel so discontent? What did you do and how did you do it? Using this as a guideline you will slowly start to bring more consciousness to sex. Being observant of the consequences of our sexual interaction is a way of bringing light into the darkness. When we are able to see the outcome of our unconscious aspects in sex, it spurs us on to transform it now with consciousness. Slowly we shine a light on something that was shrouded in mystery, bringing in the light of our intelligence.

We find this transformation through transition, the growing into a unique sexual expression through finding our way, creating experiential foundations. It is not assisted through replacing one approach with the other, high ideals, impatience, or tension. A danger lies in ruining the childlike joy and sensuality of discovering through bodily experience, with the rigidity of restriction to hide not knowing. Uncertainty, shakiness, is real and contains the seeds of growth. Using the Love Keys as guidelines will support you into an experience of love that is more simple, nourishing, and loving. These are practical suggestions to enable you to permeate your body with awareness and the experience of immediacy, which reveals sex to be a fresh and uplifting experience.

I have found one common misinterpretation made by couples in their attitude to sexual exploration. This is of making a separation between the conventional and the Tantric approach to sex. Initially the superficial difference between the two is that the first focuses on movement and orgasm, while the second embraces slowness and stillness. So couples will then decide that *this* is what it is all about. They will decide before they make love how they are going to do it. "Today, are we going to be still and silent according to Tantra, or shall we do it in the old way with movement and excitement?" Even while the value of a few minutes of stillness and silence are not to be lightly dismissed, in the long run this approach creates a division and a subsequent lack of integration within the body and psychology of each person. It reinforces our duality with a soft part and a hard part. On an energetic level, too, it becomes confusing to the poles and developing their magnetic properties is severely hindered. On one hand the genitals are being asked to be sensitive and receptive, and on the other, to be tough and demanding. This duality itself is a tension, and the true roots of consciousness cannot be planted because one step forward implies two steps back. It poses the question, which way to make love—this way or that way?—rather than allowing the body intelligence to emerge through conscious trial and error.

Tantra is not asking for your *either or,* it is asking for you in your totality. It wants your movement, your excitement, your orgasms, your stillness, your inner focus—all rolled into one, with consciousness. A complete re-education in sex is offered, which transforms your sexual energy permanently. This happens as a couple, and also on an individual level. The increased sensitivity that arises through individual consciousness remains as personal growth. Should a couple separate, each person has already benefited tremendously from the mutual process. The consciousness instilled into the penis and vagina remains even if the relationship or love affair completes itself. Consciousness is consciousness and is not dependent on external circumstances. Your next lover will sense your presence immediately. Then there becomes no other way to make love except in consciousness, because this contains everything, so much more fulfilling. Movement in meditation becomes an exquisite reality. Through union of sex and spirit, integration happens at a foundation level. But this is not a transformation that comes through separation, or through deciding which way to make love today, or as I once was told, in the mornings one way and the afternoons the other! To decide beforehand with the mind which way to make love with the body overrules the sexual integrity of the bodies, and the genitals are slow in developing their magnetic finesse.

Tantra is an invitation to make love every time with awareness and consciousness. Let the starting point always be with the intention of remaining as present and conscious as possible. That is all. It is a good start. Where it goes or how it ends up is not so important, but where *you are*, where your *consciousness is*, is the significant thing. What you do is not the concern of Tantra, but *how* you do is its focus. And the *how* is to bring awareness into sex, feeling everything as it happens second by second, to come present to whatever is in the body. And since the body contains our past, our vast personal and collective conditioning, we have to face our old habits, fantasies, and urges. We meet and embrace our desires with consciousness, but at the same time we watch what is happening at a deeper level. It's like being a witness behind the lens of a camera, watching a movie in which you are the central figure. You remain conscious of the moves being made, the shortened breath, how the sexual energy is intentionally built up to the peak experience and then released. This consciousness will automatically slow you down, bring awareness to the path, and in its generosity give you enhanced pleasure. Simply begin to playfully pay attention to the process in which you are involved. It is only through bringing awareness to everything you do that sexual energy is slowly able to transform and respond spontaneously as an expression truly rooted in the body

Another drawback in the replacement approach lies in the risk of you losing your authenticity through repressing your conditioning, and this will affect you as an individual and as a couple. Unless you transform that "how," through the awareness and consciousness, lying motionless, wide-eyed, and breathing, avoiding all excitement may work for a while, but sooner or later you are likely to find yourself yawning with an urgent need to close your eyes and sleep. The connection between the penis and vagina may even feel good, but the experience will be one lacking in challenge, not one of growing into the sex energy and surrendering to its greater intelligence, of becoming expanded and alive in it. You may start to miss the excitement, and the urge to move back into unconsciousness arises, manifesting as restlessness as you make love, wanting some action, to move, to come, to give it all up and go back to the old ways. This is to be expected. Your unconsciousness is knocking on your back door because you have denied it. You have denied where you are and imposed an idea on your sexual energy, and you are where you think you should be. The unconscious needs conscious expression and not repressive denial. It needs you to dance with it, be in transit with it, gradually transforming it into consciousness. The intention of a couple, the commitment to exploring the mystery of sex, requires a conscious dance between old and new, where encountering the unconscious elements within becomes an adventure. The process is one of repeatedly returning to consciousness, to catch the moment when one has lost consciousness or moved ahead out of the realm of the present, and keep coming back to now. The central cord is the thread of consciousness which weaves its way from awareness to being aware of lapses in awareness, back and forth like a shuttle, and through this the consciousness is strengthened, the present emerges. Simply be aware where you are when you are. As we release the accumulated tensions in sex, freeing it from a constricted path, it evolves as a changeable creative dynamic force. The key is to instill the fire of awareness, keep watching and witnessing, and slowly you will find a balance and harmony grow within.

Ordinarily the energy is going out and down and we have to bring it inward so that it can flow upward. With this inversion of sexual energy, pleasure takes on a new dimension, becoming an ecstatic full body experience, and in the core of the body itself a streaming phenomenon will begin to be felt, starting from the genitals and flowing upward toward the heart and head. At first this can be very subtle, or felt only in certain places as a glowing or tingling orgasmic cellular vibration. This streaming experience grows stronger, becoming a golden highway forging its way upward in the body. Turning inward gets easier with practice, the electro-magnetic ecstasy generated through the polarity of penis and vagina reaches upward. Through the Love Keys you can forcefully push yourself into the present. This means that your attitude is one of forceful intention; you absolutely intend to bring consciousness to your body. It is an intense shift in awareness. This intensity of presence, availability to the moment, openness to yourself and your partner, are elements that contribute to the movement of these core energies. Once relaxation is established in the sexual center, it turns upward, rising with tremendous vitality.

This is the recycling, or recirculating, of the sexual energy, which returns sparkling through the core of the body to its source in the brain. The body transforms itself into an instrument with a musical inner flute able to respond to finer and finer rhythms spiraling upward, the energy taking an ecstatic flight to penetrate the higher centers. This experience intensifies as polarity deepens, with the organs of love generating ecstatic sexual energy, and the sense of sex as a divine experience continues to grow. It is an attunement to an inner phenomenon that is riveting in its intensity, serene in its silence. As a man and a woman expand and rise in love, the inner opposing pole within each body resonates, strengthening the internal rod of magnetism, silence breaks the barrier and a miraculous melting occurs—outer man unites with his inner woman, and outer woman merges with her inner man. This orgasmic fusion of male meeting female is ecstatic love and awakens the mechanism of our inner celebration.

INSPIRATION

DROP ALL MASKS. *Be true. Reveal your whole heart; be nude. Between two lovers there should not be any secrets, otherwise love is not. Drop all secrecy. It is* politics; *secrecy is politics. It should not be in love. You should not hide anything. Whatsoever arises in your heart should remain transparent to your beloved, and whatsoever arises in her heart should remain transparent to you. You should become two transparent beings to each other. By and by, you will see that through each other you are growing to a higher unity.*

By meeting the woman outside, by really meeting, loving her, committing yourself to her being, dissolving into her, melting into her, you will, by and by, start meeting the woman that is within you; you will start meeting the man that is within you. The outer woman is just a path to the inner woman; and the outer man is also just a path to the inner man. The real orgasm happens inside you when your inner man and woman meet. That is the meaning of the Hindu symbolism of ardhanarishwar. *You must have seen Shiva: half man, half woman. Each man is half man, half woman; each woman is half woman, half man. It has to be so, because half of your being comes from your father and half of your being comes from your mother. You are both. An inner orgasm, an inner meeting, an inner union is needed. But to reach to that inner union you will have to find a woman outside who responds to the inner woman, who vibrates your inner being, and your inner woman which is lying fast asleep, awakes. Through the outer woman, you have to meet the inner woman; and the same for the man.*

Osho: **Yoga, The Alpha and Omega, Vol.10**

BIBLIOGRAPHY

Barry Long, MAKING LOVE 1 & 2 (audio tapes), available from the Barry Long Foundation International, P.O. Box 574, Mullimbimby, NSW 2482 Australia

Barry Long, LOVE BRINGS ALL TO LIFE (audio tape)

Barry Long, STILLNESS IS THE WAY, The Barry Long Foundation 1989

Osho, VIGYAN BHAIRAV TANTRA VOLS. 1& 2, The Rebel Publishing House. These two volumes were originally published as *The Book of Secrets*, Vols. 1-5 by Rajneesh Foundation International 1976. Compiled from a series of discourses given by Osho in Bombay, India between October 1, 1972 to November 8, 1973, republished in 1998 as *The Book of Secrets* by St. Martin's Press, New York (available from Osho Viha Book Distributors, PO Box 352, Mill Valley, CA 94942, U.S.A. E-mail: oshoavia@aol.com)

Osho, DIMENSIONS BEYOND THE KNOW, The Rebel Publishing House 1989

Osho, FROM SEX TO SUPERCONSCIOUSNESS, The Rebel Publishing House 1989

Osho, IN SEARCH OF THE MIRACULOUS VOL. 2, The Rebel Publishing House 1987

Osho, MY WAY OF THE WHITE CLOUD, Element Books 1995

Osho, NEW ALCHEMY TO TURN YOU ON, The Rajneesh Foundation International 1978

Osho, PSYCHOLOGY OF THE ESOTERIC, The Rebel Publishing House 1994

Osho, TANTRA – THE SUPREME UNDERSTANDING, The Rajneesh Foundation International 1975

Osho, THE TANTRA VISION VOLS. 1& 2, The Rajneesh Foundation International 1978/9 respectively

BOOKS OF RELATED INTEREST FROM NAB

BEATING TANTRA AT ITS OWN GAME : Spiritual Sexuality — *Arthur Lytle*
Tantra introduces a middle path, extending the delights of male-female coupling into rarely attained Bliss. Through integrating all levels of human consciousness, the usual short period of arousal, climax, and afterglow is extended for hours at a time without debilitation. This text lucidly discusses the 'What', 'How', and 'Why' of exercises capable of transforming sensuality and sexuality into Spirituality.

ISBN: 81-7822-148-9

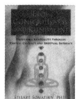

EROS, CONSCIOUSNESS AND KUNDALINI: Deepening Sensuality Through Tantric Celibacy and Spiritual Intimacy — *Stuart Sovatsky*
A superb book on kundalini yoga and its relation to both sexuality and spirituality. *Eros, Consciousness and Kundalini* is an intellectually profound and emotionally moving book. It brings to vivid, breathing life for modern sensibilities the ancient teachings of Tantric celibacy. Highly recommended.

ISBN: 81-7822-179-9

A METHOD FOR TANTRIC BLISS: The Ipsalu Formula — *Bodhi Avinasha*
A Method for Tantric Bliss presents a practical approach to spiritual awakening, leading to a joyful experience of who you really are, and your oneness with all things, your bliss. Created on a solid foundation of ancient principles and practices with deep psychological insights, The Ipsalu Formula works for everyone who practices it.

ISBN: 81-7822-189-6

TAOIST BEDROOM SECRETS — *Master Chian Zettnersan*
Learn more about the deep sexual wisdom of Love. This fascinating work focuses on the *"jade stem"* and the *"jade gate,"* which symbolize the exchange of masculine and feminine energy. The strongly vitalizing power of the many illustrated chi exercises can be recognized in names like "Return to Springtime" or "The Heavenly Water of the Life force".

ISBN: 81-7822-133-0